Integrated Behavioral Health in Primary Care

For Neftali Serrano —

Stephanie B. Gold • Larry A. Green
Editors

Integrated Behavioral Health in Primary Care

Your Patients Are Waiting

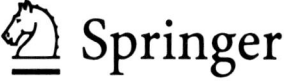
Springer

Editors
Stephanie B. Gold, MD
Eugene S. Farley, Jr. Health
Policy Center
Aurora, CO
USA

Larry A. Green, MD
Eugene S. Farley, Jr. Health
Policy Center
Aurora, CO
USA

Department of Family Medicine
University of Colorado School
of Medicine
Aurora, CO
USA

Department of Family
Medicine, University of
Colorado School of Medicine,
Aurora, CO
USA

Department of Family Medicine
Denver Health
Denver, CO
USA

ISBN 978-3-319-98586-2   ISBN 978-3-319-98587-9   (Ebook)
https://doi.org/10.1007/978-3-319-98587-9

Library of Congress Control Number: 2018957096

© Springer Nature Switzerland AG 2019
This work is subject to copyright. All rights are reserved by the Publisher, whether the whole or part of the material is concerned, specifically the rights of translation, reprinting, reuse of illustrations, recitation, broadcasting, reproduction on microfilms or in any other physical way, and transmission or information storage and retrieval, electronic adaptation, computer software, or by similar or dissimilar methodology now known or hereafter developed.
The use of general descriptive names, registered names, trademarks, service marks, etc. in this publication does not imply, even in the absence of a specific statement, that such names are exempt from the relevant protective laws and regulations and therefore free for general use.
The publisher, the authors, and the editors are safe to assume that the advice and information in this book are believed to be true and accurate at the date of publication. Neither the publisher nor the authors or the editors give a warranty, express or implied, with respect to the material contained herein or for any errors or omissions that may have been made. The publisher remains neutral with regard to jurisdictional claims in published maps and institutional affiliations.

This Springer imprint is published by the registered company Springer Nature Switzerland AG
The registered company address is: Gewerbestrasse 11, 6330 Cham, Switzerland

Acknowledgments

We are indebted to C. J. Peek, who in addition to writing Chap. 2, authored the preambles to each chapter and provided initial thought leadership and guidance on the entire book's development.

We are grateful for the assistance of our independent reviewers for their commentary and suggestions that helped make this a better book: Perry Dickinson, Bob Ferrer, John Flanagan, Bonnie Jortberg, Roger Kathol, Neil Korsen, Samantha Monson, Laura Pickler, and Ali Shmerling, Sarah Hemeida, and Lina Brou at the Eugene S. Farley Jr. Health Policy Center, University of Colorado. Thanks to Emma Gilchrist, also at the Farley Health Policy Center, for her work on Fig. 1.1 in Chap. 1.

We also wish to acknowledge the hardworking practices of the Advancing Care Together project and Integrated Workforce Study whose pioneering efforts in integrated behavioral health and primary care are the foundation of the messages delivered in this book: Axis Health System, Durango, Colorado; Bender Medical Group, Inc., Fort Collins, Colorado; Denver Health and Hospital, Denver, Colorado; Jefferson Center for Mental Health, Wheat Ridge, Colorado; Kaiser Permanente Colorado, Denver, Colorado; Midvalley Family Practice, Basalt, Colorado; Plan de Salud del Valle Inc., Brighton, Colorado; Primary Care Partners, Grand Junction, Colorado; Southeast Mental Health Services, La Junta,

Colorado; University of Colorado Aging Center, Colorado Springs, Colorado; Westminster Medical Clinic, Westminster, Colorado; Cherokee Health Systems, Knoxville, Tennessee; Edward Hines, Jr. VA Hospital – Primary Care Behavioral Health Program, Hines, Illinois; Fairview Clinics – Integrated Primary Care, Fairview Health Services, Minneapolis, Minnesota; Golden Valley Health Centers, Merced, California; Institute for Family Health, New York, New York; Penobscot Community Health Care – Summer Street Health Center, Bangor, Maine; Southcentral Foundation, Anchorage, Alaska; and Swift River Family Medicine, in collaboration with Tri-County Mental Health Services, Rumford, Maine.

Contents

1 **Why You Should Read this Book** 1
   Stephanie B. Gold and Larry A. Green

2 **What Is Integrated Behavioral Health?** 11
   C. J. Peek

3 **A Real-Life Story in Getting Started:
   Designing a Foundation** 33
   R. Scott Hammond and Caitlin Barba

4 **A Real-Life Story in Getting Started:
   Building from the Ground Up** 59
   Caitlin Barba and R. Scott Hammond

5 **Everyone Leads** 103
   Frank Verloin deGruy III and Parinda Khatri

6 **It Takes a Team** 131
   F. Alexander Blount

7 **Measure What Matters** 157
   Deborah J. Cohen
   and Bijal A. Balasubramanian

8 Where Practice Meets Policy 177
Stephanie R. Kirchner, Stephanie B. Gold,
and Benjamin F. Miller

9 Closing: It Is a Journey, Not a Destination. 203
Larry A. Green and Stephanie B. Gold

Appendix A 215

Appendix B 219

Index 245

Contributors

Bijal A. Balasubramanian, MBBS, PhD Department of Epidemiology, Human Genetics, and Environmental Sciences, UTHealth School of Public Health in Dallas, Dallas, TX, USA

Caitlin Barba, MPH Westminster Medical Clinic, Westminster, CO, USA

F. Alexander Blount, EdD Department of Clinical Psychology, Antioch University New England, Keene, NH, USA

Department of Family Medicine and Psychiatry, University of Massachusetts Medical School, Amherst, MA, USA

Deborah J. Cohen, PhD Department of Family Medicine, Oregon Health & Science University, Portland, OR, USA

Frank Verloin deGruy III, MD, MSFM Department of Family Medicine, University of Colorado School of Medicine, Aurora, CO, USA

Stephanie B. Gold, MD Eugene S. Farley, Jr. Health Policy Center, Aurora, CO, USA

Department of Family Medicine, University of Colorado School of Medicine, Aurora, CO, USA

Department of Family Medicine, Denver Health, Denver, CO, USA

Larry A. Green, MD Eugene S. Farley, Jr. Health Policy Center, Aurora, CO, USA

Department of Family Medicine, University of Colorado School of Medicine, Aurora, CO, USA

R. Scott Hammond, MD, FAAFP Westminster Medical Clinic, Westminster, CO, USA

Department of Family Medicine, University of Colorado School of Medicine, Aurora, CO, USA

Parinda Khatri, PhD Cherokee Health Systems, Knoxville, TN, USA

Stephanie R. Kirchner, MSPH, RD Eugene S. Farley, Jr. Health Policy Center, Aurora, CO, USA

Department of Family Medicine, University of Colorado School of Medicine, Aurora, CO, USA

Benjamin F. Miller, PsyD Well Being Trust, Oakland, CA, USA

C. J. Peek, PhD Department of Family Medicine and Community Health, University of Minnesota Medical School, Minneapolis, MN, USA

Chapter 1
Why You Should Read this Book

Stephanie B. Gold and Larry A. Green

Behavioral health problems spare no one, and experienced primary care clinicians know this and work with patients with these problems every day. Behavioral health problems constitute major causes of premature mortality and complicate caring for people with acute and chronic diseases of all types [1]. There is widespread agreement that primary care practices have the opportunity to improve millions of lives by improving their care of patients with behavioral health problems.

The case for changing primary care practices to integrate behavioral health and primary care is strong [2–4] (see Fig. 1.1). Not only is there a high prevalence of mental health and substance use disorders, but also low rates of patients with these

S. B. Gold (✉)
Eugene S. Farley, Jr. Health Policy Center, Aurora, CO, USA

Department of Family Medicine, University of Colorado School of Medicine, Aurora, CO, USA

Department of Family Medicine, Denver Health, Denver, CO, USA
e-mail: stephanie.gold@ucdenver.edu

L. A. Green
Eugene S. Farley, Jr. Health Policy Center, Aurora, CO, USA

Department of Family Medicine, University of Colorado School of Medicine, Aurora, CO, USA
e-mail: larry.green@ucdenver.edu

© Springer Nature Switzerland AG 2019
S. B. Gold, L. A. Green (eds.), *Integrated Behavioral Health in Primary Care*, https://doi.org/10.1007/978-3-319-98587-9_1

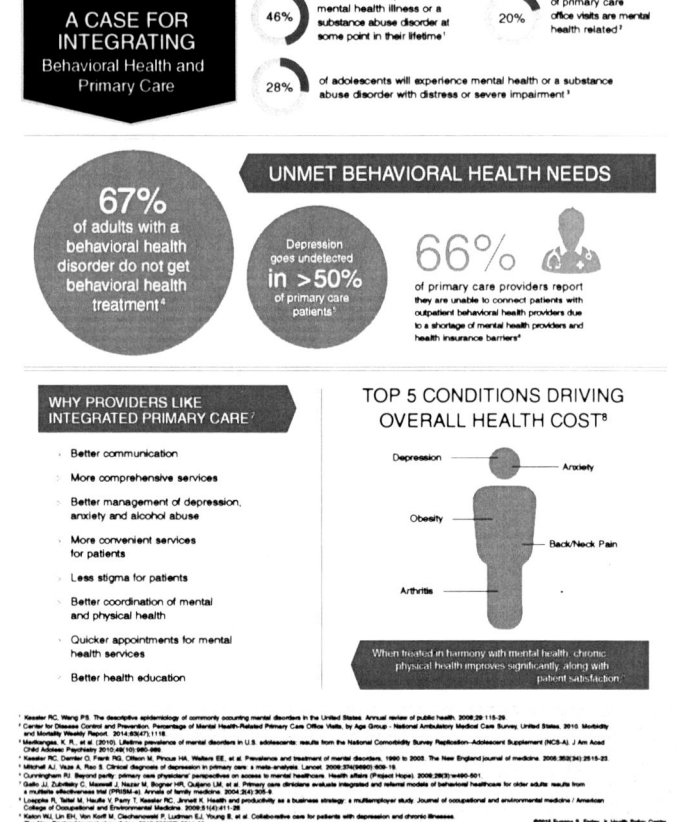

FIGURE 1.1 A case for integrating behavioral health and primary care. (Reproduced with permission from the Eugene S. Farley, Jr. Health Policy Center)

needs receiving treatment. There is a growing body of evidence that integrating behavioral health to meet these needs is feasible, reduces expenditures [5–7], and improves outcomes [8–10]. Here lies the monumental opportunity for primary care clinicians. And this opportunity is the focus of this book.

Chapter 1   Why You Should Read this Book

While many behavioral health problems can be ameliorated or resolved in primary care practices, few frontline primary care practices are fully equipped to address them. There have been a number of books written on behavioral health integration directed toward behavioral health clinicians on what they need to do to change their practice to work in primary care, but there is a paucity of practical guidance for primary care clinicians. This book aims to help fill this gap and provide information specifically for primary care clinicians who recognize that integrating primary care and behavioral health can improve their practices, the lives of their patients, and their own joy of practice.

This book is focused on pragmatic, primary care clinicians who go to work every day aiming to help their patients be healthier. It aspires to be a usable guide for regular practices wanting to take better care of their patients by improving the care of their patients with behavioral health problems. This usability is enhanced by a conversational rather than academic tone, relaying information as would be shared from one clinician to another. This conversational style, however, should not be misinterpreted as indicating a lack of evidence. The chapters purposefully blend published evidence with the real-life experience of practicing primary care clinicians who have integrated behavioral health in their practices. The ideas and principles herein are applicable to diverse patients and any primary care practice, including practices across the globe. Specific examples are used to illustrate concepts, and these particulars are specific to the United States; while the examples may not apply to other countries, the underlying concepts often have parallels in other corners of the world.

This book is also intended for practice change facilitators, practice and system administrators, and other healthcare workers seeking to transform their practices to comprehensively meet the needs of their patients *and avoid a false division of physical and behavioral health problems*. Though it is written for the local primary care team, the language often addresses primary care physicians or primary care clinicians directly—because most books on this subject have been addressed to behavioral health clinicians or large system administrators. The authors want to be sure to address the local primary care physician in the style and context in which they are familiar. Often a team leader or instigator of change within the practice, the physicians work in close partnership with their clinic manager or administrative partner and their clinical team. So if you are not a physician, please do not take offense or feel excluded when you encounter a sentence addressed straight to a doctor. It is, but it is addressed to you too—all of you who make things happen in a primary care clinic.

This book is not an exhaustive compendium of research and research methods relevant to studying care that integrates primary care and behavioral health. Neither does it delineate the diagnostic and treatment skills necessary to treat behavioral health concerns in a primary care practice. It also does not elaborate all the specific details for all of the models of integration that have been pursued. Instead, this book drills down to essentials primary care clinicians need to know and do to accomplish changes in their practice necessary to integrate behavioral health and primary care in local, real-world environments.

The chapters in this book are grounded in lessons learned and judgments made by early adopters of integrated behavioral health and pioneering change agents, educators, and evaluators. The framework of this book was derived from the insights of a group of early adopters involved in a program called Advancing Care Together (ACT) [11]. The ACT program, sponsored by the Colorado Health Foundation and administered by the Department of Family Medicine at the University of Colorado, brought together 11 primary care practices and community mental health centers in small and large, urban and rural settings across Colorado to integrate behavioral health and primary care as they saw fit. A small amount of funding was provided to support participation in the program's evaluation and learning community. After 3 years of working on integrating care, these innovators came together to share their experiences and insights. Key, hard-won messages emerged that they wanted to pass on as

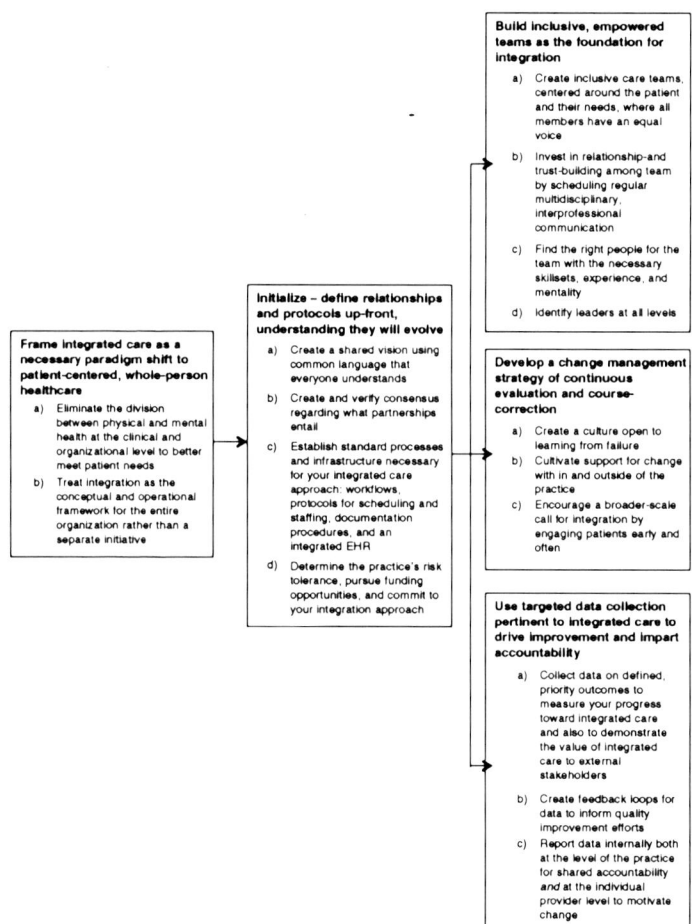

FIGURE 1.2 Lessons learned by early innovators on how to integrate care in your practice: relationships between main themes captured from participants in the Advancing Care Together study at their closing meeting, September 2014. (Reproduced with permission from the American Board of Family Medicine)

colleagues to those willing to follow in their footsteps [12]. These insights were organized and published as shown in Fig. 1.2, and this book expands on their consensus conclusions and recommendations. It is worth highlighting that these innovators recommended involving your patients early and often as you transform your practice to integrate primary care and behavioral health. After all, patients are experts in themselves.

Additional evaluations of the program from these ACT innovators and others examine the costs of integrating care [13], physical space layouts in an integrated clinic [14], adequate staffing and scheduling [15], the ways in which behavioral health and primary care clinicians interact [16], workforce preparation needs [17], electronic health record challenges and solutions [18], and the extent to which integrated services reached the target population [19]. These publications, like this book, are based in the pragmatism of practicing primary care clinicians and are freely available with many citations to relevant literature not included in this book.

Each of this book's chapter authors has years of experience in integration on the ground; together they combine the perspectives of primary care clinicians, behavioral health clinicians, practice administrators, health system leaders, primary care researchers, and practice transformation experts with concrete steps on how to make integrated behavioral health work. You may notice overlapping areas addressed in multiple chapters through different lenses; the interlocking nature of each chapter is intended to reaffirm and build upon content from other chapters and reflect the value of repetition in adult learning.

In Chap. 2, What Is Integrated Behavioral Health?, you will hear from psychologist CJ Peek about what constitutes integrated behavioral health and words and explanations you can use to make the case for integrating behavioral health to others in your practice and/or larger system. In Chaps. 3 and 4, A Real-Life Story in Getting Started: Designing a Foundation and Building from the Ground Up, family physician Scott Hammond and practice administrator Caitlin Barba tell their story together to help other primary care practices really understand integrated care, what it entails, and what it takes to do it. This story is divided into two parts to cover the candid, biographical, 25-year expedition of Westminster Medical Clinic in Colorado. Readers will understand why the following chapters dive deeper into their critical topics.

In Chap. 5, Everyone Leads, family physician Frank deGruy and psychologist and healthcare system clinical officer Parinda Khatri describe the nature and functions of *adaptive* leadership in transforming practice to integrate primary care and behavioral health. It is a function not of one person in a top-down hierarchy but of all team members. In Chap. 6, It Takes a Team, educator and psychologist Alexander ("Sandy") Blount characterizes different models of integration and explores how a team of primary care clinicians, behavioral health clinicians, and other team members can best work together to take care of patients, including strategies for hiring, communication, and developing a team culture. In Chap. 7, Measure What Matters, primary care practice researchers Deborah Cohen and Bijal Balasubramanian provide a practical framework and details about how you can measure your progress to help you make adjustments to your plans and make sure that what you do is leading to the changes you want to see. They affirm that practices do not have to measure everything that can be measured; they should measure what they need to measure so they can see how their practice is changing. In Chap. 8, Where Practice Meets Policy, psychologist and policy expert Ben Miller, practice transformation expert Stephanie Kirchner, and family physician and book co-editor Stephanie Gold characterize the importance of the larger policy environment in which your practice exists. Using current examples from the US, they describe how local policies and situations may lag behind your progress which can constrain or enable your transformation to integrated care. They limit their focus to three areas that are often problematic for primary care practices: financing integrated care, workforce issues, and getting and using the data you need to implement and sustain your approach. They explore workarounds to cope with the status quo until policies can catch up to your advances in practice. Finally, in Chap. 9, we co-editors reprise key messages to send you on your way to integrated care.

If you read this book from start to finish, you will see that the false dichotomy of physical and behavioral health is obsolete and can be replaced with a dramatically improved approach in primary care. You will be able to imagine your course toward robust, integrated primary care for whole people, grounded in evidence but most importantly in the practical realities of everyday clinical practice at the frontlines of healthcare. The whole person care that your patients are waiting for does not happen on its own. It takes commitment, leadership, collaboration, and persistence. But this journey also gives back, fostering joy in practice through working as a part of a team to provide radically improved care for many, if not most, of your patients and seeing the difference it makes in the lives of your patients and their families. Now, let us get clear about what integrated care really is.

References

1. Mokdad AH, Marks JS, Stroup DF, Gerberding JL. Actual causes of death in the United States, 2000. JAMA. 2004;291:1238–45.
2. Katon WJ, Unutzer J. Health reform and the affordable care act: the importance of mental health treatment to achieving the triple aim. J Psychosom Res. 2013;74(6):533–7.
3. Butler M, Kane RL, McAlpin D, et al. Integration of mental health/substance abuse and primary care no. 173 in. Rockville, MD: Agency for Healthcare Research and Quality; 2008.
4. WHO. The World Health Report 2001: mental health – new understanding, new hope. Geneva: World Health Organization; 2001.
5. Melek SP, Norris DT, Paulus J, Matthews K, Weaver A, Davenport S. Potential economic impact of integrated medical-behavioral healthcare: Updated projections for 2017. Milliman Research Report, January 2018.
6. Ross KM, Gilchrist EC, Melek SP, Gordon PD, Ruland SL, Miller BF. Cost savings associated with an alternative payment model for integrating behavioral health in primary care. Trans Behav Med. iby054. https://doi.org/10.1093/tbm/iby054.
7. Lanoye A, Stewart KE, Rybarczyk BD, et al. The impact of integrated psychological services in a safety net primary care clinic on medical utilization. J Clin Psychol. 2017;73:681–92.

8. Balasubramanian BA, Cohen DJ, Jetelina KK, Dickinson LM, Davis M, Gunn R, Gowen K, Miller BF, Green LA. Outcomes of integrated behavioral health with primary care. J Am Board Family Med. 2017;30(2):130–9.
9. Asarnow JR, Rozenman M, Wiblin J, Zeltzer L. Integrated medical-behavioral care compared with usual primary Care for Child and Adolescent Behavioral Health: a meta-analysis. JAMA Pediatr. 2015;169(10):929–37.
10. Archer J, Bower P, Gilbody S, Lovell K, Richards D, Gask L, Dickens C, Coventry P. Collaborative care for depression and anxiety problems. Cochrane Database Syst Rev. 2012;10:CD006525.
11. Green LA, Cifuentes M. Advancing caret together by integrating primary care and behavioral health. JABFM. 2016;28: S1–6.
12. Gold SB, Green LA, Peek CJ. From our practice to yours: key messages for the journey to integrated behavioral health. J Am Board Fam Med. 2017;30:25–34.
13. Wallace NT, Cohen DJ, Gunn R, et al. Start-up and ongoing practice expenses of behavioral health and primary care integration interventions in the advancing care together (ACT) program. J Am Board Fam Med. 2015;28(Suppl 1):S86–97.
14. Gunn R, Davis MM, Hall J, et al. Designing clinical space for the delivery of integrated behavioral health and primary care. J Am Board Fam Med. 2015;28(Suppl 1):S52–62.
15. Davis MM, Balasubramanian BA, Cifuentes M, et al. Clinician staffing, scheduling, and engagement strategies among primary care practices delivering integrated care. J Am Board Fam Med. 2015;28(Suppl 1):S32–40.
16. Cohen DJ, Davis M, Balasubramanian BA, et al. Integrating behavioral health and primary care: consulting, coordinating and collaborating among professionals. J Am Board Fam Med. 2015;28(Suppl 1):S21–31.
17. Hall J, Cohen DJ, Davis M, et al. Preparing the workforce for behavioral health and primary care integration. J Am Board Fam Med. 2015;28(Suppl 1):S41–51.
18. Cifuentes M, Davis M, Fernald D, Gunn R, Dickinson P, Cohen DJ. Electronic health record challenges, workarounds, and solutions observed in practices integrating behavioral health and primary care. J Am Board Fam Med. 2015;28(Suppl 1):S63–72.
19. Balasubramanian BA, Fernald D, Dickinson LM, et al. REACH of interventions integrating primary care and behavioral health. J Am Board Fam Med. 2015;28(Suppl 1):S73–85.

Chapter 2
What Is Integrated Behavioral Health?

C. J. Peek

Preamble

Behavioral health integration can initially mean many things to many people; the concept and its implementation can become a source of confusion for physicians and innovation teams. Clinics can reduce initial ambiguity or confusion with a good enough shared view of what behavioral health integration looks like in action—based on national definitions tailored to the local situation. As a result, clinic leaders and implementers will be much clearer about required functions they need to implement. And their patients will be clearer on what they can expect from integrated behavioral health, once implemented. *CJP*

Introduction

Behavioral health integration can mean many things to many people. This chapter aims to provide physicians (and their teams) with accurate and practical ways to answer a question

C. J. Peek
Department of Family Medicine and Community Health,
University of Minnesota Medical School, Minneapolis, MN, USA
e-mail: cjpeek@umn.edu

© Springer Nature Switzerland AG 2019
S. B. Gold, L. A. Green (eds.), *Integrated Behavioral Health in Primary Care*, https://doi.org/10.1007/978-3-319-98587-9_2

they will be asked over and over by different people at different times for different purposes:

"What *is* integrated behavioral health anyway?"

This aim is accomplished by helping a physician champion, other clinicians, and practice team members be comfortable in:

1. Citing and using a published consensus functional definition as a general basis.
2. Using a broad range of handy, concise, and entirely compatible definitions for particular audiences and purposes
3. Being able to move from a general definition to a realistically tailored local implementation

A physician champion or innovation team can retain responsiveness to published literature and definitions while proceeding realistically in his or her own real world and the people in it. While doing this could sound like a recipe for "mush" or "anything goes," this chapter offers systematic thinking on how to tailor your local work to general requirements and focus basic definitions to fit the situation at hand. This is to preserve the clinician's need to remain professionally responsible while being practical "in the moment and on the ground"—communicating well and briefly to anyone who asks.

Think about different compatible definitions for different purposes.

Part of working with definitions and being a systematic good communicator is being comfortable with a wide range of *different*, but compatible and accurate answers to "what is integrated behavioral health," not just one "best" definition. What all these definitions should have in common is being *concise*—which means (1) expressing all the important information and (2) in few words. This implies a balance between "brief" and "detailed enough."

In your communications as a clinician or leader in your clinic, you will constantly be balancing "all the important information" and "in few words." The balance you strike depends on who you are talking to and their purposes—what aspects they are interested in and how many "pixels" in the picture they need to see right then. A rule of thumb is to create short handy definitions with distillations of key elements from the *full-blown* definitions. In that way, you are not introducing a different "picture," just taking pixels out of the original picture—and you can add them back selectively as needed for different purposes while keeping the essence the same.

As you will see in Sect. 2.1, the published consensus definition (from the United States Agency for Healthcare Research and Quality, AHRQ) contains as much or more information or "pixels" that you could ever want. But it is designed so that it can be progressively streamlined or "compressed"—down to two sentences if needed. As you will see in Sect. 2.2, simply expanding or compressing a general published definition likely does not meet all your needs to answer "what is it" as asked by different people with different purposes. For this purpose, you will need a range of concise answers focused on what that person wants to know.

Use the Published AHRQ Consensus Definition as an Expandable Basis for Conversation

Published agreement exists through AHRQ [1] on what high-level functions are required to count as genuine integrated behavioral health—what it looks like in action. This is an extended consensus definition created by a panel of well-known leaders and implementers in the field. It is an excellent reference, "north star," and professional resource, even though far too detailed for most everyday conversation.

First, the two-sentence "what is it" definition (Table 2.1):

Note the broad scope of what is meant by "behavioral health" in the second sentence, far broader than diagnosable mental illnesses and conditions.

For a little more detail, use the "how" part of the definition. If you use the two-sentence definition but ask, "how do you do it," Table 2.2 shows the required functions of integrated behavioral health. This adds a few more "pixels":

TABLE 2.1 AHRQ two-sentence "what is it" definition

What is integrated behavioral health?

The care that results from a practice team of primary care and behavioral health clinicians, working together with patients and families, using a systematic and cost-effective approach to provide patient-centered care for a defined population. This care may address mental health and substance use conditions, health behaviors (including their contribution to chronic medical illnesses), life stressors and crises, stress-related physical symptoms, and ineffective patterns of health-care utilization.

TABLE 2.2 AHRQ two-sentence definition augmented with "how" and "supported by" functions

Clinical how: What integrated behavioral health needs to look like in action

1. A practice team of primary care and behavioral health clinicians tailored to the needs of your clinic panel and each patient and situation.

2. With a shared population and mission—a panel of patients in common for total health outcomes.

3. Routinely using a systematic clinical approach consisting of shared goals, workflows, and documentation.

Supported by—organizational functions taking place:

4. A community, population, or individuals expecting that behavioral health and primary care will be integrated as a standard of care.

5. Reliable office practice systems, alignment of leadership and purpose, and sustainable business model.

6. Continuous quality improvement with routine use of practice and other data to improve effectiveness.

This definition includes not only a clinical "how," but an organizational "supported by"—because the clinical methods cannot be built or sustained without these organizational supporting functions well enough in place.

Chapter 2   What Is Integrated Behavioral Health?   15

This enhancement to the two-sentence definition may be quite enough for most conversations. But at other times, you will hear, "Please be specific about what is involved." Table 2.3 shows the AHRQ definition expanded with many

TABLE 2.3 AHRQ definition with many of its clarifying sub-points

What is integrated behavioral health?

The care that results from a practice team of primary care and behavioral health clinicians, working together with patients and families, using a systematic and cost-effective approach to provide patient-centered care for a defined population.
This care may address mental health and substance use conditions, health behaviors (including their contribution to chronic medical illnesses), life stressors and crises, stress-related physical symptoms, and ineffective patterns of health-care utilization.

How: *What integrated behavioral health needs to look like in action—defining functions you need to see taking place*

1. *A practice team tailored to the needs of each patient and situation.*
   (The mix suited to serve your target population. For example, different kinds of physicians, behavioral health clinicians, social workers, consulting psychiatrists, care coordinators, clinical pharmacists, or others)
   A. With a suitable range of behavioral health and primary care expertise and role functions available to draw from. So that the team can be defined at the level of each patient and, in general, for targeted populations.
   B. With shared operations, workflows, and practice culture. Shared physical space, workflows that ensure collaboration and shared treatment plans, and unified rather than separate and conflicting medical and behavioral health practice cultures.
   C. Having had formal or on-the-job training. For both medical and behavioral health clinicians— clinical roles and relationships, culture- and team-building.

2. *With a shared population and mission*—a panel of patients in common for total health outcomes
   The patient panel and total health mission is shared by both primary care and behavioral health clinicians—not subdivided into a medical portion and a separate behavioral health portion.

(continued)

TABLE 2.3 (continued)

3. *Routinely using a systematic clinical approach* to:
   A. Identify those members of the population who need or may benefit
   B. Engage patients and families in identifying their needs for care and clinicians
   C. Involve both patients and clinicians in decision-making
   D. Use an explicit, unified, and shared care plan in a shared electronic medical record
   E. Systematically follow up and adjust treatment plans if patients are not improving as expected ("treat to target") (The presence and routine use of these systematic clinical processes is a defining marker for integrated behavioral health)

Supported by — **organizational enabling functions taking place**

(The team and clinical functions above are far less likely to take place sustainably without these organizational supports)

4. *A community, population, or individuals expecting behavioral health and primary care to be integrated* as a standard of care (sometimes referred to as "patient demand").
   A general standard of care, not just a localized enhancement or featured program in otherwise separated medical and behavioral health work.

5. *Office systems, alignment of leadership and purpose, and sustainable business model*
   A. Clinic operational systems and office processes consistently support interprofessional communication, shared care plans, tracking care, and other collaborative functions.
   B. Leadership, supervision, and incentives are aligned to support the functions of integrated behavioral health.
   C. The business model sustains integrated behavioral health (or is working toward that end).

6. *And continuous quality improvement and measurement of effectiveness* (to know what is working or not)
   A. Routinely collecting and using practice-based data to track and improve patient outcomes, change what the practice is doing, and quickly learn from experience.
   B. Periodically examining and reporting outcomes — at the clinician and program level — for care, patient experience, and affordability ("Triple Aim") to engage the practice in making changes accordingly.

of its clarifying sub-points. That many "pixels" are likely required for conversations about implementation — "what do I have to build exactly?"

The published AHRQ definition includes much more than you see in Table 2.3, should you need it, e.g., elements of a shared integrated behavioral healthcare plan and elements of systematic follow-up and adjustment of treatment. It has a table of contents with links, with more detail than you probably ever want to know.

The AHRQ definition is not the only useful resource. For example, the SAMHSA-HRSA "Standard Framework for Levels of Integrated Healthcare" has a structure you can adapt in the same way — starting with a one- or two-sentence definition and adding specifics or "pixels" to the picture as needed [2].

But there is more to having a broad repertoire of handy answers to "what is it" than compressing or expanding the AHRQ or other published definitions. You will likely need handy definitions for the needs and concerns of particular audiences and purposes.

Have a Range of Handy Answers to "What Is It" for Particular Audiences and Purposes

A clinician or other practice leader will be asked the "what is integrated behavioral health" question in all kinds of situations by all kinds of people with different purposes and different need for detail. So you will want a range of different, but entirely compatible answers or "definitions" tailored to different people and purposes. Having concise and contextually appropriate answers to "what is integrated behavioral health" can be regarded as a leader function that is open to all — as described in Chap. 5.

Table 2.4 offers examples of equivalent definitions or answers for different persons commonly encountered in the primary care environment. Because these persons have different purposes in asking the question, the answers are different, but equally accurate and almost equivalent. The content within all these sample responses can be found within

TABLE 2.4 Compatible answers to "what is it" for different audiences and purposes

Person asking	Likely purpose	Sample answer
Physician colleague	Just interested in what you are trying to do	Expanding our clinic team to do better (and feel better) with the behavioral health dimension of our practice…things our patients already bring with them…that we may not always have the time or experience to do as well as we want. "The care you want to provide to your patients."
Clinic nurse or medical assistant	How will this affect my routine and who I work with?	A BH clinician on our clinic team instead of an outside referral… works in clinic space with you and is part of huddles, care planning, and charting…on our team like everyone else…helps patients and helps us.
Operations team	What operational changes to expect?	A BH clinician working on our team from empty exam rooms, offices, or other clinic space…in our huddles, scheduling and EHR systems…coding…picture on the wall with the rest of us…another role on our primary care team.
Clinic manager	What supervision and business model?	Licensed BH provider with own professional supervision but accountable to us (medical director and clinic manager) for teamwork, citizenship, scheduling, care processes…revenue for codes when appropriate, indirect benefit to clinic performance, and [fill in the rest of your business model].

Quality improvement leader	What is the QI opportunity?	Take your pick: Integrated BH processes for 1. Better clinical outcomes for BH conditions 2. Better outcomes for medical or complex conditions where people are depressed, demoralized, anxious, or "stuck" 3. Quicker initial access to BH consultation for patients (and for us) 4. Better connection for any specialty BH referrals 5. Better patient and provider satisfaction 6. Reduced fragmentation and needless cost of care 7. Realistically tailoring medical care to accommodate "social determinants" and "complexity"
Patient	How might this help me?	Your doctor has a partner right in the clinic trained to help our patients with personal, family, stress-related, mental health, or healthy behavior kinds of factors in health and medical care…a stronger medical team when you need it…Right here in the clinic… Where we all know each other.

(continued)

TABLE 2.4 (continued)

Person asking	Likely purpose	Sample answer
Board member	How might this affect our mission, reputation, and viability?	Our mission is to improve health. BH is also health—Often intertwined with medical conditions and care. We are implicitly "scored" on BH contributors to good primary care via clinical outcomes, patient experience, cost of care, and provider satisfaction. For these reasons, BH integration has broad national uptake. Research and business models are still in development, but BH integration as a normal part of primary care is pretty much settled. The task is how to do it effectively. We know what the functions need to be.
Implementation or process design team	What exactly do we have to build?	Read the AHRQ functional definition (Table 2.3) and go to the published lexicon for other specifics such as the list of elements for shared care plans and elements for follow-up and treatment to target. These are essential functions, but still do not tell us exactly what to do here. So consider how we can tailor these functions to our own practice, at the time we are beginning, at the pace we can move, with our own target starter populations, and with the resources and tolerance for change around us.

the AHRQ definition, but is translated for use by the person and purpose at hand.

These are only examples. You can tailor your own responses that could be given between floor 1 and 2 on an elevator. But they could be followed with "Would you like to know more about that?" This would open the path for another layer of information for anyone interested—such as in Tables 2.1, 2.2, and 2.3 showing the AHRQ definition.

Be Able to Move from General Definitions to Your Own Locally Tailored Implementation

The AHRQ definitions of Tables 2.1, 2.2, and 2.3 or person-specific examples in Table 2.4 do not try to prescribe a specific granular implementation for your practice. There is too much to take into account locally to make any universal detailed prescription realistic. Just as a great definition of "airliner" does not include the mechanical drawings for any specific airplane, the functional definition of integrated behavioral health does not include exactly what to implement in your own clinic. Yet the need remains for a specific implementation that works for your purposes.

Some implementers employ a "model of integration" to help tie general definition to specific implementation. A "model" is simply one of the currently recognized ways to operationalize the functions required in a general definition. Operating models are different means to the same or similar ends, but represent different distinguishable ways to "skin the cat" in different settings. Hence conversations about "what is integrated behavioral health" sometimes include the question, *"What models of integration are out there and should I use one of them?"*

It is worth pausing here to briefly describe common "models" that people may have heard about. Read Table 2.5 as a general guide, knowing that the terminology and specifics within these models are variable, evolving, and entail considerable overlap. For example, the first two models in the table (Primary Care Behavioral Health and Collaborative Care

TABLE 2.5 Common operating models of behavioral health integration

Common name(s)	Basic approach
1. Primary Care Behavioral Health (PCBH)	Characterized by BH clinicians as on-site members of the primary care team, space and EHR; doing brief interventions using more or less standard algorithms. Degree of standardization, length of intervention, or clinical focus varies [4–7].
2. Collaborative Care Model (CCM)	Defined by a team of primary care provider, care manager, and consulting psychiatrist who reviews registry panels of patients and consults to care manager, PCPs, and other clinical staff of the care team. The psychiatrist is an active consultant, not there to fill a conventional schedule of patients. Often involves considerable standardization and has a long history of research support [8–12].
3. Primary care integrated in mental health settings (bidirectional or "reverse integration")	Primary care clinician expertise brought into mental health settings so that patients who identify mainly with the MH clinic get good primary care right there. This model aims for much of the same functional performance as integration of MH into PC [13, 14].
4. Residency behavioral science education model	Almost universal in family medicine residencies, a behavioral health clinician works as teacher, preceptor, and clinician seeing patients with physicians—already on-site for educational purposes. Pulls in elements from the PCBH model but rhythms, schedules, and scope of activities are different due to being educational programs.
5. Behavioral health integration in specialty medical care	Similar goals and functions as primary care integration but tailored to specialty medical care such as oncology, neurology, endocrinology, occupational health, physical medicine and rehabilitation, developmental pediatrics, or emergency department and hospital. May use a combination of PCBH, CCM, or residency education models.

TABLE 2.5 (continued)

Common name(s)	Basic approach
6. Family-centered integration or medical family therapy	The family is considered the "client" and recipient of medical care. Family systems are front and center with identified patient embedded in a family system where much of the causality and treatment or self-management opportunities reside. Many principles of PCBH or CCM integration apply, but with the family rather than individual as the "client" [15].
Other variations or hybrids	Specific implementations may combine elements from more than one model above or employ telehealth and other variations on collaboration for rural or other special circumstances.

Model) are sometimes featured independently as anchoring models and sometimes are combined in actual implementations. In academic settings such as family medicine residencies, one or both may be combined with the "residency behavioral science education" model.

Models are a package of design choices. Here are some important things to remember about "models":

1. *Models are shorthand for particular approaches* to accomplishing the same core functions—a pattern of design choices. For example, the Collaborative Care Model archetypically features a primary care physician, care manager, and consulting psychiatrist collaborating using a registry for "treatment to target" for one or more conditions.
2. *Models often emerge from different research or practice cultures.* For example, the Primary Care Behavioral Health model emerges from clinical practice culture, typically aimed at a wide variety of patient conditions and situations ("all comers"). The Collaborative Care Model emerged from a research culture (originally on late-life depression) and has gradually been extended to multiple conditions.
3. *Different models may be chosen based on practicalities*—what or who is available to do the work, and what operational or information systems are available. For example,

the Collaborative Care Model might be difficult to implement in an area with no psychiatrists, or none willing to work as consultants to primary care providers.
4. *All "models" are a means, not an end.* They must accomplish the same basic functions of the AHRQ definition or equivalent general definitions. There is little point in arguing about "which flavor of integrated care" is best [3]. Each model has its own origins and properties, but they tend to mix and converge over time. Keep your eye on the defining functions of integrated behavioral health and "models" as a means to achieving them.

Fidelity to a model or definition also requires realistic local tailoring, whether designing an implementation using a *model* of integration as a pattern, or working directly from the general *definitions*, to work…

…in your own practice,
…with what you can gather around you at the time you begin,
…at the pace you can move,
…with your own target starter populations and purposes, and
…with the resources and tolerance for change around you.

Implementing integrated behavioral health on a meaningful scale requires a definition or model to be scaled up (a pattern to be followed) and local tailoring (making it work well in local reality). There is value in both, and tension between "standardization" and "anything goes" does not go away. These are the characteristics of "polarities" requiring that you strike a balance between them [16–23].

Balance means preserving the *general case* while creating a local *special case*; the *essence* of the definition and what *within it* needs to be locally adapted. And do not leave that balance to the imagination. Actual implementation requires a shared understanding at a practical level of detail on what requires fidelity and what is locally tailored. Let us consider two examples of local tailoring to a specific *model* of integration.

Example 1

The DIAMOND Initiative was a Minnesota statewide initiative for care of depression following the Collaborative Care

Model (CCM), with a care manager and consulting psychiatrist working with primary care providers[1] [12, 17, 22, 24]. Especially because it had to be scaled up to 75 practices statewide, it was essential to be clear what components were essential—the core features—and what aspects of those components the practices had to do or decide for themselves. DIAMOND required fidelity to four components:

1. A stepped care protocol
2. A registry for all DIAMOND patients
3. A care manager working with primary care clinicians, patients, consulting psychiatrist
4. A consulting psychiatrist

These were all required to participate in DIAMOND. Clinic training materials included highly specific definition of those four components plus specifically what the clinics would need to build or adapt to their own situations.[2] Here are a few examples of what every practice did:

- Tracked a certain set of data, but the type of medical record or tracking system was up to the practice.
- Had a dedicated care manager trained by the project, but the discipline was up to the practice, e.g., nurse, social worker, behavioral health clinician, medical assistant.
- Received a care management fee, but each practice negotiated its own rate with payers.

The required functions and what was to be locally decided were made explicit at the outset to minimize confusion across the 75 practices and to prevent both "cookie cutter" prescriptions that would exclude many practices, and so much diffusion of the intervention by "local tailoring" such that "anything goes."

---

1 The DIAMOND Initiative (Depression Improvement Across Minnesota, Offering a New Direction) was a cooperative effort of 75 practices from small and large provider groups, supported by a financial model from all four major health plans and the Minnesota Dept. of Human Services, and facilitated by the Institute for Clinical Systems Improvement, a regional quality improvement organization.
2 DIAMOND fidelity/local tailoring examples were extracted by the author from training materials supplied to all practices.

Example 2

Local tailoring can be done directly to a functional definition of integrated care without an intervening model. The AHRQ "lexicon" definition of integrated behavioral health does not entail or recommend a "model" such as CCM or PCBH. Table 2.6 shows a worksheet that can be used by your practice to help your implementation team be clear about what your clinic(s) can and must decide or do for yourselves given your local situation. Of course, this worksheet still does not actually tell you what you are going to do. But the "local tailoring" column asks the questions for which you will need answers. You can fill in those specific answers—which would begin to sketch out your own "special case" of integrated behavioral health.

TABLE 2.6 A worksheet for balancing fidelity with local tailoring for integrated behavioral healthcare

Defining functions: what must be in place—fidelity	**Local tailoring: choices you need to make**	**What specifically you will implement**
Clinical "how" functions:		(Write it down here)
1. A practice team of primary care and behavioral health clinicians tailored to the needs of your clinic panel and each patient and situation With shared space, workflows, treatment plans, and practice culture	• The mix of clinical skills and experience needed for your clinic's panel or target sub-population for integrated behavioral health • Your processes for defining the team at the level of each patient, and targeted population • Your particular space and workflows that ensure teamwork in a single, not conflicting practice culture • How you orient and train clinicians for roles	

TABLE 2.6 (continued)

Defining functions: what must be in place—fidelity	Local tailoring: choices you need to make	What specifically you will implement
2. With a shared population and mission—a panel of patients in common for total health outcomes Not merely separate responsibility for separately conceived medical and behavioral health	• How you help your clinicians make this cultural shift and get used to thinking of medical and behavioral health both as "health" and "whole person care" • How you make sure interests, incentives, and trust are aligned ("leadership alignment")	

3. Routinely using a systematic clinical approach consisting of shared goals, workflows, and documentation	Your specific processes for:
	  • Identification of those who can benefit
	  • Engaging them in integrated behavioral health
	  • Involving them in decision-making
	  • Making shared care plans in your EHR
	  • Systematic monitoring, follow-up, and treatment adjustment ("treat to target")	

(continued)

TABLE 2.6 (continued)

Defining functions: what must be in place—fidelity	Local tailoring: choices you need to make	What specifically you will implement

Organizational "supported by" functions

4. A community, population, or individuals expecting that behavioral health and primary care will be integrated as a standard of care	How you engage your patients, community groups, provider societies, and local health groups in establishing this as a target standard of care or "north star" in your community	
5. Reliable office practice systems, alignment of leadership and purpose, and sustainable business model Broad-based visible organizational support for what it takes to do integrated behavioral health	• How you reach durable leadership consensus — and align the incentives and reasons • How you will redesign processes to support the functions • The financial workarounds to support the work before standard payment supports it well enough	
6. Continuous quality improvement with routine use of practice and other data to improve effectiveness Track and improve patient outcomes, change and quickly learn from experience. Triple Aim	• How you expand your quality improvement tracking to reflect the integrated behavioral aspects of care, not only medical—a more integrated "scorecard" • How you will report results and use it to improve the integrated system, not only traditional medical outcomes	

Conclusion

This chapter has been a long answer to the question, "What is integrated behavioral health?" All practice leaders and implementers may need to answer this in one or more of the three ways outlined here:

1. What is integrated behavioral health in general (a published, professionally grounded definition—the general case)?
2. What does that mean for me here? (Handy context-specific answers to the "what is it" question for various audiences and occasions)
3. How specifically will we make it work with who we are here? (The locally tailored implementation that you will be creating in your own clinic.)

With these three ways to answer *"what is it,"* your team can retain responsiveness to published literature and definitions while proceeding realistically in your real-world situation with the people in it; preserving the need to remain professionally responsible, *and* be practical about implementing things in the local context, *and* communicating well and briefly to anyone who asks.

References

1. Peek CJ and the National Integration Academy Council (2013). Lexicon for Behavioral Health and Primary Care Integration: Concepts and Definitions Developed by Expert Consensus. http://integrationacademy.ahrq.gov/lexicon.
2. Standard Framework for Levels of Integrated Healthcare. Center for Integrated Health Solutions, SAMHSA-HRSA. http://www.integration.samhsa.gov/resource/standard-framework-for-levels-of-integrated-healthcare
3. Unützer J. Which Flavor of Integrated Care? Psychiatric News. 2014;49(20)

References for PCBH model

4. Reiter JT, Dobmeyer AC, Hunter CL. The primary care behavioral health (PCBH) model: an overview and operational definition. J Clin Psychol Med Settings. 2018 Feb;26:109. https://doi.org/10.1007/s10880-017-9531-x.
5. Vogel ME, Kanzler KE, Aikens JE, Goodie JL. Integration of behavioral health and primary care: current knowledge and future directions.J. Behav Med. 2017;40(1):69–84. https://doi.org/10.1007/s10865-016-9798-7.
6. Beehler GP, Lilienthal KR, Possemato K, Johnson EM, King PR, Shepardson RL, et al. Narrative review of provider behavior in primary care behavioral, vol. 35. How Process Data Can Inform Quality Improvement. Fam Syst Health: Health; 2017. p. 257. https://doi.org/10.1037/fsh0000263.
7. Funderburk J, Dobmeyer A, Hunter C, Walsh C. Provider practices in the Primary Care Behavioral Health (PCBH) model: an initial examination in the Veterans Health Administration and United States Air Force. Families, Sytems, & Health. 2013;31(4):341–53. https://doi.org/10.1037/a0032770.

References for CCM model

8. The University of Washington AIMS Center. https://aims.uw.edu/collaborative-care
9. Unützer J, Katon W, Callahan CM, Williams JW Jr, Hunkeler E, Harpole L, Hoffing M, Della Penna RD, Noël PH, Lin EH, Areán PA, Hegel MT, Tang L, Belin TR, Oishi S, Langston C. Collabrative care management of late-life depression in the primary care setting: a randomized controlled trial. JAMA. 2002;288(22):2836–45.
10. Katon WJ, Lin EH, Von Korff M, Ciechanowski P, Ludman EJ, Young B, et al. Collaborative care for patients with depression and chronic illnesses. N Engl J Med. 2010;363(27):2611–20. https://doi.org/10.1056/NEJMoa1003955.
11. Bauer AM, Azzone V, Goldman HH, Alexander L, Unutzer J, Coleman-Beattie B, Frank RG. Implementation of collaborative depression management at community-based primary care clinics: an evaluation. Psychiatr Serv. 2011;62(9):1047–53. https://doi.org/10.1176/appi.ps.62.9.104710.1176/ps.62.9.pss6209_1047.

12. Solberg LI, et al. The DIAMOND initiative: implementing collaborative care for depression in 75 primary care clinics. Implementation Science. 2013;8:135.

References on integration of primary care in mental health settings ("reverse integration")

13. Maragakis A, Siddharthan R, RachBeisel J, Snipes C. Creating a 'reverse' integrated primary and mental healthcare clinic for those with serious mental illness. Prim Health Care Res Dev. 2016 Sep;17(5):421–7. https://doi.org/10.1017/S1463423615000523.
14. Gerrity, M., Zoller E. et al. Milbank memorial fund. Integrating primary care into behavioral health settings: What works for individuals with serious mental illness. 2014. https://www.integration.samhsa.gov/integrated-care-models/Integrating-Primary-Care-Report.pdf

Reference to medical family therapy

15. McDaniel S, Doherty W, Hepworth J. Medical Family Therapy and Integrated Care (second edition). Washington, DC: American Psychological Association; 2014.
16. Barry Johnson (1992). Polarity management: identifying and managing unsolvable problems. HRD Press. See also www.polaritymanagement.com.

Literature relevant to fidelity and local tailoring:

17. Crain AL, et al. Designing and implementing research on a state-wide quality improvement initiative: The DIAMOND study and initiative. Med Care. 2013;51(9):e58–66.
18. Fleuren M, et al. Multiple determinants of innovation adoption. Int J of Quality Health Care 16:107–23.
19. Callahan CM, et al. Implementing dementia care models in primary care settings: The Aging Brain Care Medical Home. Aging Ment Health. 2011;15(1):5–12.

20. Kitson AL, et al. Evaluating the successful implementation of evidence into practice using the PARiHS framework: theoretical and practical challenges. Implementation Science 2008;3:1. https://doi.org/10.1186/1748-5908-3-1
21. Stroebel CK, et al. How complexity science can inform a reflective process for improvement in primary care practices. Jt Comm J Qual Patient Saf. 2005;3198:438–46.
22. Solberg LI, et al. Partnership research: a practical trial design for evaluation of a natural experiment to improve depression care. Med Care. 2010;48(7):576–82.
23. Crabtree BF, Miller WL, Stange KC. Understanding practice from the ground up. J Fam Pract. 2001;50(10):881–7.

DIAMOND

24. Solberg LI, et al. A stepped wedge evaluation of an initiative to spread the collaborative care model for depression in primary care. Ann Fam Med. 2015;13:412–20.

Resources

In addition to providing definitions and frameworks, these two organizations provide a package of resources for integrated behavioral health:

The AHRQ Academy for Integration of Behavioral Health and Primary Care: https://integrationacademy.ahrq.gov

The Substance Abuse and Mental Health Services Administration – Health Resources and Services Administration (SAMHSA-HRSA)'s Center for Integrated Health Solutions: https://www.integration.samhsa.gov

Chapter 3
A Real-Life Story in Getting Started: Designing a Foundation

R. Scott Hammond and Caitlin Barba

Preamble

After "what is integrated behavioral health," the question of "how to do it" quickly emerges. But this does not begin by cutting straight to changes in workflows and protocols. It starts with a foundation for success—a shared vision of integrated behavioral health in our practice, medical and behavioral health partners with shared goals, and steps to merge different practice cultures and language. This means deep conversation with medical and behavioral health colleagues on what we want to be and do together—knowing that "colleagues" means not only clinicians of different disciplines but also practice managers and staff. Standing together on this foundation creates starter conditions for making change—and is a case example exemplifying the content of the rest of this book. *CJP*

R. S. Hammond (✉)
Westminster Medical Clinic, Westminster, CO, USA

Department of Family Medicine, University of Colorado School of Medicine, Aurora, CO, USA

C. Barba
Westminster Medical Clinic, Westminster, CO, USA
e-mail: caitlin.barba@westminstermedicalclinic.com

Introduction

Westminster Medical Clinic (WMC) was first opened in 1952 and remains a small, physician-owned family medicine practice serving approximately 6000 patients in a northwest suburb of Denver, Colorado. Our payer mix is 70% commercial, 25% Medicare Advantage and Medicare B, and 5% uninsured. WMC has been a National Committee for Quality Assurance (NCQA) recognized Patient-Centered Medical Home, Level 3 since 2009. Our team care is structured after the Bodenheimer Teamlet Model [1]. Our core team consists of a physician, one to two midlevel clinicians and two to three medical assistants supported by an RN care manager, care coordinator, 1.5 FTE behavioral health professionals, a certified health coach, and a chiropractor. WMC has participated in numerous pilots, grants, and initiatives since 2003. In 2013, following a rigorous nationwide search, WMC was selected as 1 of 30 exemplar practices by the Robert Wood Johnson Foundation and the MacColl Center for Health Care Innovation at the Group Health Research Institute to participate in the Learning from Effective Ambulatory Practices (LEAP) project. More recently, the clinic participated in Advancing Care Together, the State Innovation Model, and the Comprehensive Primary Care Plus initiative.

> *"One thing hastens into being*
> *Another hastens out*
> *Even while a thing is in the act of*
> *coming into existence*
> *Some part of it has ceased to be*
> *Flex and change are forever renewing the*
> *fabric of the universe*
> *Just as the ceaseless sweep of time is forever*
> *renewing the face of eternity*
> *In such a running river where*
> *there is no firm foothold,*
> *What is there for man to value*
> *Among all the many things that are*
> *Racing past him."*
> Marcus Aurelius, Meditations 6:15

RSH On a typical, hectic day, I paused at the door. My patient was waiting to see me for a routine chronic care visit. I planned on how to navigate the appointment with the myriad of checklists, measures, and tasks to address. My eyes focused on what was written on his one-page intake form. It broke the concentration from my regimented chart review; he checked feeling down and not sleeping well. At that moment, I closed my eyes and took a long, deep breath to reframe our visit together.

Immediately, tears ran down his face when I asked him how he was doing. My planned visit was no longer the priority; the person sitting in front of me was. The air in the room was still and emotionally charged, as he needed patience and compassion. After some sensitive probing, I said, "I think it best we discuss your diabetes at another time. You are doing okay. Would you rather discuss what is troubling you today?" It was clear that he was in crisis and a brief intervention followed. He needed immediate help and I asked, "I would like to introduce you to Dr. Allison, who can see you right now. Is that okay with you?"

The right care was provided with the right person, in the right place, and at the right time. This was our vision. As medicine evolves into genomics, transcriptomics, proteomics, and metabolomics to treat disease with remarkable precision, we must also remain patient-centered to support healing relationships through the traditional values of medicine. Personomics [2], the knowledge of the patient as a person in their community, encompasses the National Institute for Health and Clinical Excellence (NICE) guidelines [3]. These guidelines include knowing the patient as an individual; understanding their life circumstances, concerns, specific needs, and perspective; and avoiding making judgments or assumptions based on their appearance or characteristics. Since the social determinants of health, including their epigenetic expression [4], affect an individual's susceptibility to disease and response to treatment, these concerns must be addressed to truly target the patient's unique biologic variability and provide personalized, whole-person care.

Medicine, and primary care in particular, is subject to incessant changes and great demands that are both exciting and exhausting simultaneously. In the United States, behavioral healthcare has been disconnected from medical care for many reasons. Unfortunately, mental illness knows no boundaries and this fragmentation has led to significant gaps in care. This division of care is antithetical to the teachings of Hippocrates who first systemized medicine and recognized that the brain is the seat of consciousness. He dispelled the notion of demonic possessions and superstition as the cause of mental illness stating, "mental illness is treated more effectively if handled in a similar manner to physical medical conditions" [5]. He outlined the common bond of all healers to observe critically; treat the patient, not the disease; evaluate your diagnosis and treatment honestly; and assist nature. These principles are our professional roots and continue to be relevant today to restore a "healthy mind in a healthy body" [6].

History is the soul of man and illuminates the foundational values of medicine. In our chaotic healthcare system, as Marcus Aurelius queried, "what is there for man to value?" To fuel our passion to persevere and to serve as the standard for our actions, we incorporated the contemporary values of medicine—respect for autonomy, beneficence, non-maleficence, and justice [7]. In this river of constantly changing and expanding information, these medical principles and contemporary core values were our firm foothold *among all the many things racing past us* and soothed us in the uncomfortable, and, at times, painful process to adapt, evolve, and stay true to the Hippocratic directives.

Pragmatically, designing the foundation for integration requires a clear shared-vision, strong defined partnerships, efficient operations and protocols, and a sustainable program. Over time, we unknowingly followed the ancient wisdom of Lao Tzu, "To be ready for success, first fail" [8]. Our initial attempts to integrate behavioral health into primary care failed for several reasons. Initially, we reacted to fulfilling a need, not following a vision, and were driven by a passion to provide whole-person care without the supporting infrastructure. We felt the urgency to abandon the status quo but we were not clear on exactly why nor did we understand the dynamics and operational structure of team care.

It took many years for our clinic to develop the resources, mindset, teams, and heart to reach this place. In that context, we will take a personal and conversational approach to share our journey and what we have learned. With these reflections on how to avoid certain obstacles, we offer a perspective of our experience, both physician and practice manager, in the belief that the path to behavioral health integration is the product of this collaboration to lead and facilitate change together.

We hope to engage you as an active reader with strategic questions and exercises to help clarify your vision, needs, and resolve to successfully reach your goals. Knowing stops when questions cease. Solving a problem may not be so much in finding the answers but in asking the right questions [9]. Asking the right questions helps you unlearn many assumptions that create barriers and helps you see the critical issues from different perspectives to move from thought to action.

Integrating behavioral health is more than a journey; it is an expedition of discovery with a specific purpose and destination. You may be starting or, as we did a few times, restarting your journey. We acknowledge your course will not exactly mirror ours as your professional and personal circumstances are unique. We operate from the bias of a small, independent, private practice, but our transformational process is universal and can be adapted to any organization.

Constructing Your Vision with Personal Reflection

> "Your vision will become clear only when you can look into your own heart.
> Who looks outside, dreams; who looks inside, awakes."
> Carl Jung

RSH The journey began in 1993 and could not have started under more arduous circumstances as I took one breathless step after another at 19,000 feet. Similarly, at altitude, one slow thought follows another in this mindful, existential alpine environment bringing a clarity not easily found in normal daily activities. Vision quests are common to all cultures and this was mine. Rising above the jungle landscape in Ecuador, Cotapaxi (19,347 feet/5897 meters) presents a challenging and dangerous climb. One week prior to our arrival, ten climbers perished in an avalanche on a neighboring peak. I took this trek with my best friend who was a licensed clinical social worker and inclusive thinker. We shared many mutual patients that were subject to the siloed, disconnected healthcare system. On simple, rugged paths and around camp stoves under glittering, cool night skies, we pondered over life and purpose as middle-aged men do. Here and on other treks, we solidified the direction we needed to take to fulfill our pledge as healers and it was together on a path with heart.

It was a handshake deal. No contract or arrangement of how to work together other than a common goal and a few additional operations for staff to maintain. We stumbled into in a rudimentary form of team care that lasted for a few years, ultimately, failing due to this lack of legal and operational structure.

A few years later, in a second attempt to integrate, the clinic contracted with a local mental health organization, but this relationship faltered because we did not have a clear understanding of each other's needs and neither of us had a vision for why, what, and how we were going to provide care in a sustainable way.

More years passed and we were on our own doing "our best" to provide the behavioral health needs of our patients with the insufficient time and resources available to primary care. The numerous and varied demands and expectations of patients and the profession took priority. It was in 2003 when I stumbled across the Chronic Care Model [10] and I understood why my training (acute care medicine) did not work in practice (acute/chronic/prevention care). As a result, we began engaging in quality improvement projects in earnest. Finally in 2008 with the release of NCQA's Patient-Center Medical Home model [11] coupled with the Institute for Healthcare Improvement's Triple Aim [12] in 2009, I understood the full scope of primary care within a framework of the structured elements for team care.

Hubert Humphrey said, "The moral test of government is how it treats those at the dawn of life – the children; those at

Chapter 3 A Real-Life Story in Getting Started

the twilight of life – the aged; and those in the shadows of life – the sick, the needy, and the handicapped." These moral directives were embedded in the PCMH, and I was excited to finally have a blueprint to outline our responsibilities and expectations. What was missing was more intangible. Workflow, infrastructure, measures and the like certainly promote efficient and effective care; however, as in climbing, the purpose and drive to reach the peak is personal.

The same is true in creating visions in medicine. A vision is different than the catchy and memorable slogans designed to capture one's attention. To create a vision, you must first inventory your personal values and beliefs and combine them with your past experiences to conceptualize what needs to change, what you want to achieve, and for whom. Without this introspection, one is doomed to follow someone else's vision that may or may not be aligned with your own.

> *Strategic Questions #1*
> *– Questions you should ask to create your personal vision:*
> *What is your current scope of care? Ethically, what care should be given to patients?*
> *What are your core values?*
> *Is your current work in line with your values?*
> *What motivates you?*
> *What is the patient experience you want to create?*
> *What are possible ways to accomplish what you believe the future should be?*
> *What are your assets? Limitations?*
> *What can be realistically achieved in your setting or system?*
> *What are your boundaries? What are you willing to compromise to achieve your vision? What must you preserve?*

If I could reverse time, knowing that a concrete vision is necessary for integration success, I would have pursued a personal exploration to define this vision at the beginning. It took 25 years to shape cloudy and idealistic ideas into a specific and practical vision that was both achievable and sustainable [13].

> *Westminster Medical Clinic seeks to provide exemplary, high-quality, and accessible primary care within a healing environment. We believe in the enduring values of medicine —sharing in*

decision-making (respect the autonomy of the patient); practicing in the best interest of the patient (beneficence); providing safe care (non-malfeasance); ensuring honesty, fairness, and equality in care (justice); and promoting provider and staff well-being (harmony).[1]

Exercise #1
To formalize a concrete vision to share, write down your specific responses to Strategic Question #1. Read it today, next week, and in 1 month. After each reading, expand your responses into how this vision will look, feel, and sound on a daily basis with staff and patients. How does this vision reflect your personal journey? Will it achieve what you want to accomplish for the patient and for the practice?
Share your evolving vision with others in the practice (partner-owner, providers, administrator) to plant a seed and gauge if your ideas resonate with your team and intersect with current gaps in care. Intentionally sharing your vision is described in the next section.

Vision and mission statements often blur; however, it was clear to us that only by addressing all the medical, physical, and behavioral health needs of our patients could we realize this vision and achieve a mission that both reflects our core competencies and outlines our goals:

> *Our Mission is to provide comprehensive, coordinated, and personalized, whole-person care and work with the community to support healthier living.*

Visions may change, expand, or retract over time depending on where the future leads. In our case, I wanted to ensure that we identified and treated the behavioral health needs of all of our patients. This mini-vision comfortably fit into our mission. Once your vision and mission are clearly established, the next step is to lead your team to make the future now with behavioral health integration as a priority.

---

1 In 2012, WMC added the Quaternary Aim, physician and staff well-being to the Triple Aim (IHI). Bodenheimer and Sinsky later coined the term, Quadruple Aim https://www.ncbi.nlm.nih.gov/pmc/articles/PMC4226781/. In 2017, we adopted the Quintuple Aim (Frank Reed, M.D. communication) to create a competitive business advantage for employers since businesses provide over 50% of healthcare coverage in the USA.

Sharing your Vision through a Guiding Coalition

CB I had a serious childhood illness that lasted 12 painful years. Physicians and hospitals were safe places that gave me hope, no matter the content of the visits. I always believed in the possibility of a better tomorrow, even if it was not remission. As for many stricken with an illness, my experiences required a new frame of mind and resilience that shaped my enduring belief that anything is possible. I developed an appreciation for the nature of healing relationships between clinicians and patients and learned that "healing, as opposed to curing, gives us a sense of meaning in hardship and hope in suffering." [14]

Healing is a transformational process from intervention to outcome, touching on the physical, mental, emotional, spiritual, familial, social, communal, and environmental dimensions of illness that does not focus only on the disease but on the person [15]. People look for healing in many places and ways. This journey may support or hinder the healing process. What a paradox for patients when they have difficulty accessing behavioral health from their trusted primary care clinician who does not provide this fundamental healing opportunity. Although I found my own way through my chronic illness, I know I could have benefited as an early adolescent from whole-person, comprehensive care.

I would not have guessed that my background in mathematics, in conjunction with my personal experience with the healthcare system, would lead to an administration and managerial-leadership role at a clinical practice. My strength in developing systematic steps to reach an end, combined with my compassion and desire to help the suffering, steered my decision and interest to impact health on a population level.

To work in primary care as a manager, a master's degree in public health fit my personal goals better than a degree in health administration or business administration. Although there is overlap across the degrees, I was educated to manage community health initiatives, program design, and apply quality improvement philosophy to healthcare delivery. This training directs the main focus of care delivery to be patient-centered and supports the traditional values of medicine. I found my calling to imagine, share, and work toward creating a healing environment in primary care by using my training and experiences to share my vision. This was my path with heart.

RSH Change does not happen just because it is a good idea, and people will not follow just because you are passionate about that idea. You must research, study, and learn not only how to construct a vision but also how to share your vision. Three distinct, concurrent transitions had to occur to share my vision: manager into leader, employees into teammates, and hierarchical organization into collaborative team care [16].

The first step is to find a manager who has the personal drive for excellence beyond a desire to just do a good job, as well as the openness to explore a new working relationship with the physician-leader. Managers have the daunting task to support, inspire, and cultivate the vision while managing a plethora of daily operations. One needs to blend the strengths of the clinician with the manager to create a leadership dyad. The ability to combine systems thinking with organizational skills creates a collaborative team capable of solving complex problems. This leadership team results in a unique and synergistic relationship that can produce remarkable results and high performance. In some ways, this is the first integration you need to achieve in your practice. In climbing, when you "rope-up" you have a heightened sense of responsibility and determination to safely reach your goal. Your partner's interest and your interest are one. Decision-making is shared. Communication is clear. Success depends on both of you. Integration of leadership lays the foundation for teambuilding in the practice and the subsequent integration of behavioral health. [17]

Exercise #2
To find a leader to manage your practice, ask:
1) What is a current health or healthcare delivery problem and why? Why is this issue important to you?
2) Why do you want to work in healthcare?
3) As a manager, what do you believe is your scope of responsibilities and how do your education and experience support you?
4) How do you lead as a manager?

5) What is your concept of teams, teamwork, and team care?
6) How do you define and measure excellence? How do you personally exhibit "excellence"?

To create a physician–manager dyad and transition from manager to leader, you must share why and how you constructed your vision. To literally get on the same page, I shared articles, books, presentations, and podcasts that inspired or shaped my vision in order to facilitate a common direction through mutual understanding. We met regularly each week to share perspectives of the teaching. Many of the references listed in this chapter were part of our "book club."

The second step is to create a guiding coalition [18], a diverse group committed to the vision and led by your manager. You must prepare your coalition to be the ambassadors that spread the vision among the clinicians and staff. This step lays the foundation to create collaborative teams by aligning values and purpose within the practice. Begin with leading the coalition in open-ended discussions focusing on why and how this vision will meet their personal goals and aspirations. In our experience, we found that the main reasons that resonate with clinicians and staff to pursue integration are increasing health equity, defragmenting physical-behavioral healthcare, improving quality of care, increasing meaningfulness in patient interactions, decreasing workflow barriers, and reducing workforce burnout through better patient access to behavioral health.

A best practice to promote sharing a vision is to clarify messages and then practice delivering those messages in different scenarios. Michael Roberto in a lecture series, The Art of Critical Decision Making, states that you must frame your vision as an opportunity and advantage as opposed to a risk or burden [19]. Your vision must be shared, dissected, and validated by each clinician and staff member to overcome the complacency that maintains the status quo [20]. This process leads to a shared commitment and shared vision. Over time, staff will also interact with patients using the same messages framed from these conversations.

The physician champion, who has one foot in the present and one foot stepping into the future, must also listen to the clinicians and engage them by linking the vision to their purpose and by showing them how the vision fulfills their clinical goals and resonates with their personal aspirations. In a study in 2009, only 14% of employed physicians felt their values aligned with leadership [21]. Clinicians are most engaged when they see their own personal gaps in care. We conducted a PCMH practice self-assessment, a Clinical and Community Needs Assessment to identify gaps in care, and shared clinician performance measures to fuel the desire to improve. During our team meetings, we discussed the clinician's role and scope of care in this vision and how this changes their clinical practice. Some felt sadness noting that integration resulted in less medical clinician-based behavioral health counseling. It took honest, sensitive conversation to accept that although they enjoy this connection, ultimately, integrated teams provide better care. As in any grieving process, leadership must help the clinician accept change and process through the denial–anger–bargaining–depression–acceptance stages of loss [22]. Integration results in other areas of clinician role changes/losses that need to be addressed. More details on leadership are explored in Chap. 5.

The third transition involves building a collaborative team of employees. Teambuilding will also be discussed in detail in Chap. 6. Briefly, we learned that all staff must participate in transformation; otherwise, it will fail. To involve the staff, we listened to their desires and needs. They were given the permission and responsibility to "work for the patient, not for the provider." Staff were encouraged to refer to patients as "our patient," not "your patient" when discussing care with providers. In workflows, they each had the authority to stop the "production line" at any sign of a quality-care issue [23, 24]. They understood that their actions could save a life and they embraced this responsibility with the cautious enthusiasm that this role demands.

This strategy reoriented our hierarchy from vertical to horizontal leadership. In other words, we changed the culture on how we worked together by transforming into a team-based organization and committing to the vision and details of implementation together.

Strategic Questions #2
What current factors need to change? What drives change or quality improvement in your practice? What support do you and your staff need?

CB Focus your attention on your *people* and *environment*. Michael Roberto continues, "Our environment shapes how we think, how we interact with those around us, and how we make judgments." Moreover, Steven Johnson in Where Do Good Ideas Come From [25] shares the importance of environment as it promotes innovation. He identifies one reason to explore good ideas is to become more innovative. He asks, "What are the spaces that have historically led to unusual rates of creativity?" Good ideas lay dormant and are not a sudden inspiration but rather occur when there is a collision of an idea with another idea(s) to mingle and become a breakthrough (even if it takes a few years). We found our guiding coalition was fertile ground for such co-mingling of ideas and provided a clear direction to guide, align, and inspire action among all clinicians and staff. Other venues to co-mingle ideas were all-staff meetings, wellness activities and retreats, and teambuilding topic-conversations.

Once teams were formed, staff needed inspiration from leadership. Inspiring action began with permission to "be the change that you want to see."[2] We instilled the belief that the vision is possible by de-escalating fears and addressing concerns. Small groups and one-on-one conversations work best. I took each staff member out to coffee or tea over 3–4 months to build on an existing relationship and to proactively ask questions, to gather ideas on improving the initial vision, and to assess their readiness to change or go through the integration journey together.

Strategic Questions #3
How can you determine if you have the right clinicians and support staff for your integration journey?

A second method of asking questions and gathering feedback came in the form of mandatory reflection homework and story writing. The question was posed to each employee: Why is behavioral health integration important to you? Much like the wide range of perspectives in the blind men and the

---

[2] Attributed to Mahatma Gandhi and paraphrased from "…If we could change ourselves, the tendencies in the world would also change. As a man changes his own nature, so does the attitude of the world change towards him…"

elephant parable, all the responses recognized the value of integration but from different viewpoints depending on how they interfaced with the patient. Our front desk personnel believed what is important to our patients is important to us. Many expressed how important it was to have behavioral health here where it is immediately available rather than making a referral. Our nurse and medical assistants wanted to have the ability to help people right away, feeling that it made a big difference since many of our triage calls are about behavioral health issues. Our Physician Assistants, who see patients with behavioral health issues every day, felt a sense of relief from overcoming the barriers to access. Everyone had a different reason or purpose for working at our clinic. You must nurture each individual's passion to make transformational change. The common denominator was that we all agreed that this was our responsibility because the majority of behavioral healthcare is delivered by primary care [26] and access to treatment presents significant barriers to patients [27]. Unlike the fragmented visions in the blind men and the elephant parable, this process of telling one's story helped establish a common reality to see the "big picture" by putting all the parts of integration together in one tangible, cohesive vision.

We had to change how we engaged one another to transform into a collaborative team. We discovered we had the right clinicians and staff. Through one-on-one coffee dates and essays, sharing "Dr. Hammond's vision" changed to "our WMC vision."

Choosing and Being Chosen as a Partner

> "If you want to travel swiftly, travel alone. If you want to travel far, travel together."
>
> African proverb

RSH Not until 2012 did our clinic have another opportunity—*Advancing Care Together*—to partner with behavioral health. In this grant, we were able to breach two major barriers to behavioral healthcare—location and cost—by co-locating a behavioral health clinician (BHC) into our practice and providing the initial six visits at no cost. We dramatically increased our reach and showed significant improvement in depression markers with positive trends in diabetes management. When the grant ended, so did the funds and this project.

After 3 years of growing and refining behavioral health integration, our BHC became an indispensable, deeply rooted team member and we could not imagine practicing without this support. We understood the value, mastered the workflow, and saw the results. We made the critical decision that we must find a way to make it work as an essential core service in our practice.

To continue with a fully integrated model, the options we considered were to employ a BHC; to co-locate with a self-employed BHC; to contract with a telepsychiatry service; or to merge services with a Community Mental Health Center. We evaluated each of these options from financial and operational perspectives within the framework of the PCMH principles. We used the comparison table below as a checklist to compare the different integration models, the strengths and weakness of applicants, and likelihood of financial viability. The clinical needs may be different for your organization. Use this worksheet to determine which model works best for your organization. Examples that applied to our practice are listed in the first row (Table 3.1).

An external partnership with a Community Mental Health Center best fit our vision, mission, and needs without the burdensome economic pressures that would threaten success. It fulfilled our mission to engage with the community as a Community-Centered Medical Home and provided access to full-service psychiatric care. Although employing our own BHC would have advantages, the clinical benefits of partnering with a Community Mental Health Center outweighed the loss of control and direction in our situation. After all, integration is a journey in collaboration.

CB We sought an external partner who shared a common vision and commitment to continue this integration journey. As Winston Churchill said, it takes courage to listen. With what we learned from previous attempts, our first step was to meet and listen to the leaders of the Community Mental Health Center to explore collaboration. To find the right fit, we first needed to be sure that we could work together through aligned values, and second, to ensure that we could satisfy the clinical needs of the practice.

Even if financial analysis is not how you primarily reach decisions, a financial plan (discussed in Chap. 4) must first be addressed before you can start exploring the details of any type of partnership. As opposed to a zero-sum game, to create a positive-sum outcome and a mutually beneficial agreement with any partner, one must satisfy the needs, desires, expectations, and interest of both parties through integrated or interest-based bargaining [28].

The fixed opinions of positional bargaining will only lead to ineffective compromise and the inability to reach an agreement. Both parties must take an honest interest in each other's needs, concerns, and desires to help mitigate against financial loss in working together. Since financial benefit is unlikely, success requires acknowledging and accepting the value of other economic and noneconomic advantages.

Assuming a financially viable model was achievable, we set out to find a Community Mental Health Center partner. We called our county mental health center first since the organization serviced our community. We did not know why an organization would want to partner with a small, private practice. How would we know if the organization was interested in partnering for integration? So, we asked.

We found that Community Mental Health Centers have the basic desire to outreach and partner with the community and recognize the barriers to behavioral health access. It was just a matter of whether they saw the value and had the resources to connect with primary care. Rick Doucet, CEO of Community Reach Center, also a participant in the *Advancing Care Together* initiative, had a strong commitment to collaborate with community partners. He accepted integration as a

TABLE 3.1 Worksheet to match PCMH principles of care and organizational needs to behavioral health clinician partnership options

PCMH principles of care	Clinical needs	Community mental health center partnership	Independent group partnership/out-sourcing	Employment
Comprehensiveness	Trained in various therapeutic styles to meet diverse patient needs (mental illness, substance abuse, chronic disease, etc.)	For example ✓ (Likely trained in various disciplines)	For example ± (Possibly trained in various disciplines)	For example ± (May need further training if no primary care experience)
	Psychiatrist backup for complex cases	✓	±	✗
	Continued education for medical providers	✓	±	✗ (Limited funds to allocate time)

(continued)

TABLE 3.1 (continued)

PCMH principles of care	Clinical needs	Community mental health center partnership	Independent group partnership/out-sourcing	Employment
Coordination	Access to specialty psychiatric care			
	Access to community resources			
	Effective, shared communication and care plans			
Whole-person orientation	Provide first contact, continuous care in all stages of life			

Accessible	Timely routine visits
	Timely urgent intervention including warm-handoffs
	24/7 emergency access
	Alternate backup when BHC unavailable
Safety, quality	Evidence-based, effective interventions applicable to population needs
	Participate in periodic measurements
Personalized	Foster an ongoing relationship with medical team and patient
	Willingness to change/ vision for change

loss leader, observed that integration is local, and invested accordingly to be successful. He acknowledged that starting with a grant is helpful, but you need to find creative ways to keep costs down to be sustainable. One must be prepared to endure a long learning curve and have the willingness to work together. He states that integration is not a plug-and-play project; you cannot duplicate the same process from practice to practice. All of the clinicians of the medical practice must demonstrate interest in working with the BHC to commit to providing whole-person care.

Daniel Fishbein, PhD, the Vice President of Corporate Business Development at Jefferson Center for Mental Health has integrated with over 30 primary care practices in metro Denver. He recommended that you search for signs on an organization's website indicating whether they are open to integration. Look for a dedicated person who is responsible for integration and has current partnerships with primary care in the community. In partnership, he states that both must satisfy the needs, desires, and expectations of one another in a mutually beneficial agreement and nurture the relationship through meetings, conversation, and a go-to person.

Experience from Physician Health Partners, a Denver management service organization, demonstrated that timing is important. If either a Community Mental Health Center or the primary care practice is going through leadership change or restructuring, collaboration is unlikely to be successful.

> *Strategic Questions #4*
> *What do you need to know to assess if a potential Center may be a good partner?*
> *1) What are your mission and long-term goals? What is your philosophy of care?*
> *2) What is your current practice culture? How do you view primary care and what is the role of primary care in behavioral health?*
> *3) What is your understanding of integration? Where are your gaps in care?*
> *4) Is the leadership willing to commit to this project, and how will they engage and support staff in this effort?*
> *5) Do they have the time and communication channels to make this successful? Do they have a dedicated employee with responsibility to manage integration initiatives in the community?*
> *6) Do they have the administrative and financial resources to integrate?*

After numerous meetings in exploring a partnership with the Community Mental Health Center, we began merging cultures to start doing the work of integration.

Merging Cultures with Behavioral Health

"Change is scientific; progress is ethical."
Bertrand Russell

"Though the leaves are many, the root is one."
William Butler Yeats

RSH Two distinct cultures, medical and behavioral health, have evolved [29]. Merging these cultures was the most challenging aspect of this transformation. Culture is the social behavior and norms developed from the knowledge, experience, beliefs, values, attitudes, and meanings acquired by a group of people or organization. Culture determines a group's vision, strategy, infrastructure, and governance policy that translates into how decisions are made and work gets done. You must respect that diversity and those differences. Although you need to preserve each other's cultural identity; ultimately, you need to create a new "we" through shared goals and shared tasks. Merging cultures is not just creating a balance between different groups. It is an evolution to a new homogenous and harmonious team.

Language and communication were our biggest challenges. Over the years, we found differences in jargon led to uncertainty in goals and relationships. Resistance to share bidirectional information and care plans led to ambiguity in assigning responsibility resulting in fragmentation of treatment. Differences in workflow expectations led to friction. Different definitions of successful outcomes resulted in misunderstanding, while different paces in practice led to a dys-synchrony in care delivery.

Strategic Question #5
How do you work together and communicate with others in patient care?

Anticipating these issues prior to our next attempt at integration and through the collaborative efforts of WMC,

Advancing Care Together, and the Colorado Center for Primary Care Innovation,[3] we developed a Compact to serve as a Rosetta Stone [See Appendix A] to bridge these differences and to create team care by providing a framework for better communication and safe transition of care between primary care and BHCs. This agreement served as a portal to a new merged culture encouraged by shared leadership and supported by definitions for integrated behavioral healthcare, types of transitions, and relational elements with primary care.

The Compact is a multidimensional tool that provides a platform for a common vision and strategy to begin a partnership and merge cultures. During the building phase, it provides an agenda and concrete plan to close critical gaps and build a collaborative team. When differences arise, it serves as an arbitration tool based on common goals and agreement. It distinguishes the sacred differences that support each other's personal identity that must be preserved when merging cultures.

Daniel Fishbein, Vice President of Corporate Business Development at Jefferson Center for Mental Health, noted that the Compact helped shift from hierarchal leadership to collaborative leadership and encouraged a "go with the flow" attitude. Many clinicians have difficulty in sharing patients and need to decrease their territorial tendencies to be responsible for all aspects of patient care. The Compact encourages a collegial relationship with the BHC, helping them become a respected and valued member of a multidisciplinary team and make the transition from a behavioral norm of episodic care to the continuity model of primary care.

CB The Compact provided solutions to the many barriers to forming functional, communicative clinician teams. The four domains of collaborative care in the Compact are: transitions of care, access, collaborative care management, and patient communication. Referral and transition of care templates are provided to ensure each clinician had the necessary

---

[3] A 501(c)3, nonprofit foundation founded by individuals at Westminster Medical Clinic

information to improve bidirectional communication and clarify responsibility and accountability.

Creating examples of ideal consult reports and providing feedback by editing initial patient consult reports helped the BHCs understand the medical language and learn the best format to provide useful information to the clinician. Similarly, the Compact provided a referral template from clinician to BHC containing the essential information to optimize the patient's first visit.

The Compact was eventually re-named *Collaborative Guidelines* to promote teamwork and partnership. The principles were easily agreed upon, but operational details required a deep-dive review and discussion with management. Several meetings followed to discuss details of scheduling, referrals, documentation of visits, sharing of visit documentation, and shared resources to provide integrated care. Details of these considerations and tips for integration are discussed in the next chapter, Building from the Ground Up.

Conclusion

To successfully implement behavioral health into primary care, you must have a clear vision and mission supported by strong values in order to withstand the distractions and misdirection of the healthcare system and overcome the inherent challenges of transformation. Building a strong team who shares this vision is paramount before integrating behavioral health. Selecting the right partner with common vision and values is critical to create the shared culture needed to achieve integration that serves the needs of both behavioral health and primary care.

There is nothing extraordinary about our practice that successfully took us down this path. We are just ordinary people who use the work of extraordinary minds. All practices have the potential for integration when vision meets determination.

References

1. Bodenheimer T, Laing B. The Teamlet model of primary care. Ann Fam Med. 2007;5:457–61.
2. Ziegelstein RC. Personomics. JAMA Intern Med. 2015;175(6):888–9.
3. Patient experience in adult NHS services: improving the experience of care for people using adult NHS services. National Institute for Health and Care Excellence. 2012. https://www.nice.org.uk/guidance/cg138/chapter/1-Guidance - tailoring-healthcare-services-for-each-patient.
4. Notterman DA, Mitchell C. Epigenetics and Understanding the Impact of the Social Determinants of Health. Pediatr Clin North Am. 2015;62(5):1227–40.
5. Ivanovic-Zuvic F. Epistemological considerations about medicine and mental health in ancient Greece. Rev Chil Neuropsiquiatr. 2004;42(3):163–75.
6. Kleisiaris C. Health care practices in ancient Greece: the Hippocratic ideal. J Med Ethics Hist Med. 2014;7:6.
7. Beauchamp T, Childress J. Principles of biomedical ethics. New York: Oxford University Press; 2001.
8. Tao Te Ching: 81 Verses.
9. Green T, Woodrow P. Insight and Action - How to discover and support a life of integrity and commitment to change. New Society Publishers. Philadelphia, PA. 1994.
10. The Chronic Care Model. Improving chronic illness care, Group Health Research Institute http://www.improvingchroniccare.org/index.php?p=The_Chronic_CareModel&s=2
11. Patient-Centered Medical Home (PCMH) Recognition. National Center for Quality Assurance. http://www.ncqa.org/programs/recognition/practices/patient-centered-medical-home-pcmh
12. The IHI Triple Aim. Institute for Healthcare Improvement. http://www.ihi.org/Engage/Initiatives/TripleAim/Pages/default.aspx
13. Beauchamp T, Childress J. Principles of biomedical ethics. New York: Oxford University Press; 2001.
14. Optimal Healing Environments: Your Healing Journey. Samueli Institute. 2013. http://www.samueliinstitute.org/File%20Library/Health%20Policy/YourHealingJourney.pdf
15. Firth K, et al. Healing, a Concept Analysis. Global Adv Health Med. 2015;4(6):44–50.
16. DeMent J. Managers, leaders, and teams in a team-based environment. Hosp Mater Manage Q. 1996 Aug;18(1):1–9.

17. Healthcare Executive. The dyad leadership model: four case studies. 2017; 32(5):32–40.
18. Kotter J. Leading Change. Boston: Harvard Business Review Press; 1996.
19. Roberto, M. The art of critical decision making. Course Guidebook; 2009.
20. Kotter J. Leading change. Boston: Harvard Business Review Press; 1996.
21. Linzer M. Working conditions in primary care. Ann Intern Med. 2009;151:28–36.
22. Kübler-Ross, E. (2005) On grief and grieving: finding the meaning of grief through the five stages of loss, Simon & Schuster Ltd. New York, NY 10020
23. Sorin T, Faul F. Lean management – the Journey from Toyota to healthcare. Rambam Maimonides Med J. 2013;4(2):e0007.
24. Joosten T, et al. Application of lean thinking to health care: issues and observations. Int J Qual Health Care. 2009;21(5):341–7.
25. Johnson S. Where good ideas come from: the natural history of innovation. New York: Riverhead Books; 2010.
26. Wang P, et al. Twelve-Month Use of Mental Health Services in the United States. Arch Gen Psychiatry. 2005;62:629–40.
27. Cunningham PJ. Beyond parity: primary care physicians' perspectives on access to mental health care. Health Affairs. 2009;28(3):490–501.
28. Spangler B. "Integrative or interest-based bargaining." Beyond Intractability. Guy Burgess and Heidi Burgess (editors). Conflict Information Consortium, University of Colorado, Boulder. Posted: June 2003.
29. Rainey L. Integrated Care: Working at the Interface of Primary Care and Behavioral Health. Washington, DC.: American Psychiatric Publishing; 2015. p. 18.

Resources

Safety Net Medical Home Initiative
http://www.safetynetmedicalhome.org/change-concepts/organized-evidence-based-care/behavioral-health
http://www.safetynetmedicalhome.org/sites/default/files/Behavioral-Health-Integration-Resources.pdf
Primary Care Team Guide.
http://www.improvingprimarycare.org

Good To Great: why some companies make the leap and others don't. Collins Jim. HarperCollins Publishers, Inc. 2001

The Improvement Guide: A Practical Approach to Enhancing Organizational Performance. Langley G et al. Jossey-Bass. 1996.

Leading Change. Kotter John, Boston. Harvard Business Review Press. 1996.

Chapter 4
A Real-Life Story in Getting Started: Building from the Ground Up

Caitlin Barba and R. Scott Hammond

Preamble

The foundation is ready and you are now able to stand on it together. But how will the "walls and roof" go up incrementally in a way that builds momentum while reflecting the shared vision? What are the tasks and a practical "construction sequence"? How are the inevitable balances struck between competing priorities within that shared vision? How can your financial plan balance revenue and noneconomic benefits? How do you balance the use of "workarounds" with more mature and sustainable methods beyond your direct control? How will you orient and train staff—and get organized to change workflows and track expected outcomes? *CJP*

Westminster Medical Clinic (WMC) was first opened in 1952 and remains a small, physician-owned family medicine practice

---

C. Barba (✉)
Westminster Medical Clinic, Westminster, CO, USA
e-mail: caitlin.barba@westminstermedicalclinic.com

R. S. Hammond
Westminster Medical Clinic, Westminster, CO, USA

Department of Family Medicine, University of Colorado School of Medicine, Aurora, CO, USA

© Springer Nature Switzerland AG 2019
S. B. Gold, L. A. Green (eds.), *Integrated Behavioral Health in Primary Care*, https://doi.org/10.1007/978-3-319-98587-9_4

serving approximately 6000 patients in a northwest suburb of Denver, Colorado. Our payer mix is 70% commercial, 25% Medicare Advantage and Medicare B, and 5% uninsured. WMC has been a National Committee for Quality Assurance (NCQA)-recognized Patient-Centered Medical Home (PCMH), Level 3, since 2009. Our team care is structured after the Bodenheimer Teamlet Model [1]. Our core team consists of a physician, one to two midlevel clinicians, and two to three medical assistants supported by an RN care manager, care coordinator, 1.5 FTE behavioral health professionals, a certified health coach, and a chiropractor. WMC has participated in numerous pilots, grants, and initiatives since 2003. In 2013, following a rigorous nationwide search, WMC was selected as 1 of 30 exemplar practices by the Robert Wood Johnson Foundation and the MacColl Center for Health Care Innovation at the Group Health Research Institute to participate in the Learning from Effective Ambulatory Practices (LEAP) project. More recently, the clinic participated in Advancing Care Together, the State Innovation Model, and the Comprehensive Primary Care Plus initiative.

Introduction

Life is a series of pulls back and forth.
You want to do one thing,
but you are bound to do something else ...
"A tension of opposites,
like a pull on a rubber band.
And most of us live somewhere in the middle."...
So which side wins?
He smiles at me, the crinkled eyes, the crooked teeth.
"Love wins. Love always wins."

Mitch Albom [2]

CB You have a vision. You have a partner. You have built a culture and a team of clinicians and support staff ready for integration. You have worked *on* your practice. Now, you and your team need time to work together and evolve *in* your practice to create a strong foundation and to support making sound decisions. No matter the size of your organization, behavioral health integration takes time, more time, and then more time. Behavioral and physical health in primary care have been separated for years. It is imperative to form realistic expectations for how long this journey will take to reconnect these two disciplines. Although it seems overwhelming at times, you can succeed when fueled by your vision, directed by a clear plan and driven by a step-by-step approach.

You can reach your vision by taking small steps over time. Integration success is not defined by one implementation step, one moment, one choice, or one lucky break. Jim Collins writes that "an overall accumulation of effort in a consistent direction" [3] generates momentum. With each implementation step, we gathered momentum and achieved our vision through patience, heart, and perseverance to attain our goal of comprehensive, whole-person patient care.

The Gantt chart below displays the categories of steps to take after you accomplish constructing and sharing a vision, partnering, and merging cultures as discussed in Chap. 3. Your organization, however, may be subject to different care delivery models, nuances in management styles, unique local legislation, and varying capacities needed to successfully integrate. Nevertheless, certain tasks must first be achieved before proceeding to the next step. The *Tasks, Tips, Questions, and Considerations* below provide topics to explore in getting started. I will outline the steps that worked for us and highlight some of the activities that supported our integration (Fig. 4.1).

Decision Priorities and Needs Assessment

There is nothing worse than a sharp image of a fuzzy concept.
Ansel Adams

CB First and foremost, I needed to determine what drives my decision-making in order to stay focused on one "side of the rubber band." Do not allow decisions to "live in the middle"; otherwise, you will lose momentum and clarity. Your

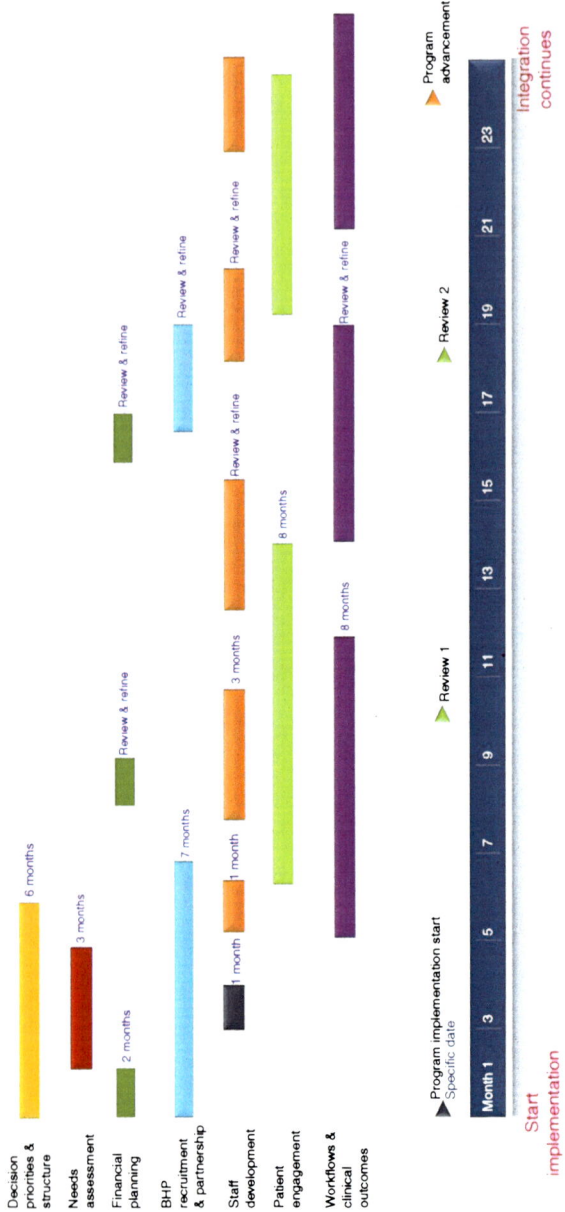

FIGURE 4.1 Gantt chart displaying an implementation timeline for behavioral health integration

TABLE 4.1 Tips, questions, and considerations for assessing clinical needs and business logistics for your integrated approach

Tasks to complete	Tips, questions, and considerations
Complete a clinical and community needs assessment	Complete prior to sharing a vision and choosing and being chosen as a partner (see Chap. 3). It is important that providers and staff know the gaps in care Review the clinical literature to select a type of therapy or model to be used in practice. The preferred model should match the needs of your population and inform a job description for a behavioral health clinician (BHC)
Review anti-kickback/Stark laws with your legal team	What is the structure of your business? Local laws, the financial relationship with a partner, and your organizational structure may impact referral patterns between medical and behavioral health
Develop a Business Associates Agreement with a Community Mental Health Center and include protected health information	Become familiar with state laws, federal laws, and HIPAA compliance. This will result in more productive discussions about expectations in documentation, continuity of care, and in sharing records with your BHC partner. This would also be relevant for practices hiring their own BHC and in clarifying relationships when external referrals are indicated

decision drivers should be embedded in your vision, mission, and your organizational values. Examples of drivers that should be measurable and attainable are quality, profits, affordability, and clinical evidence.

After determining your drivers, next, prioritize. We made a decision to offer behavioral health integration not because it would add revenue to the clinic but because it resonated with why the clinic exists and fulfilled our goal to provide comprehensive whole-person care. This reason for behavioral health integration gave us permission to plan for financial sustainability with a breakeven or loss leader strategy. You may have many drivers, but determining the primary driver as the priority will release the tension from being "bound by something else," such as health plan measures, large healthcare organization regulations, or by the most powerful force, the status quo. Instead, what binds you can be your patients and their needs.

There are various methods of identifying community needs. Use a needs assessment template or asset-based mapping materials to get started.

First, assess the needs of your local community. State and county public health departments and the Centers for Disease Control share population-level data of health indicators in your area. Identify the medical conditions and social determinants of health in your geographic area. In our state, diabetes is most prevalent in our county.

Second, gather population data on your established patients. Run a report in your electronic health record (EHR) to determine the most frequently documented diagnosis codes. When we began behavioral health integration, our list of 10–20 most frequent codes included diabetes, hypertension, pain, and acute issues. Over time, depression joined the list. The number of patients diagnosed with depression and anxiety will grow in the initial months of integration. The list will help assess current needs in your population. Revise the count of patients with each diagnosis on your list and review the depression and anxiety literature to estimate the number of established patients with potential behavioral health needs per diagnosis.

Third, insurers mandate clinical quality measures in various programs and initiatives. Which National Quality Forum (NQF) measures are you following? Clinical quality measures from insurers or Accountable Care Organizations may dictate who and what you measure. For example, NQF #0418 relates to the percentage of patients screened for depression with, if positive, a follow-up plan documented on the date of screening. What are your practice's or health plan's NQF clinical quality goals? Of the patients identified with the most frequently used diagnoses in Step 2, how many of those patients should be included in the denominator to meet this goal? You may also find a sub-group of patient needs in the problem lists of your patient charts. See Chap. 7 for further details on the use of measures in quality improvement.

Steps 2 and 3 both determine baseline demand for a BHC and the visits needed per day for patient access. In the next section, I will show you an example on how to use this information.

Finally, offering an anonymous patient survey gathers feedback about healthcare issues important to patients. Design survey questions to determine how patients access care and for what reasons patients seek care. Ask patients if they would use a BHC located in your practice and gather reasons for why or why not. Patient feedback also creates a list of reasons and conditions why patients who do not have a Diagnostic and Statistical Manual of Mental Disorders-V (DSM-V) diagnosis want to see a BHC. This is important since billable services are linked to DSM-V. Adjust the patient count from Steps 2 and 3 earlier to equal a final estimation for patient demand per day that accommodates all needs in the practice.

Based on your population's acceptance of BHC counseling and the practical skill set of your clinicians to treat behavioral health conditions, you will also need to determine the best clinical model of care (Solution-Focused Brief Therapy (SFBT), Cognitive-Based Therapy, others) that will improve the health outcomes of the populations you have identified in the needs assessment and that are preferred by your medical providers. This will require input from your physician champion. As in many practices, our providers frequently medically manage patients and voiced a great desire to access psychiatrists for medication consultation; consulting psychiatrists are a prominent feature of some integrated models, such as the Collaborative Care Model or TEAMCare.

RSH From a provider perspective, the overall needs were easy to identify since we live the gaps in care on a daily basis. Our barriers to care included limited time to adequately screen and evaluate behavioral health symptoms and limited access to behavioral health services. Our patients struggled with financial issues and the fear and anxiety of obtaining care at unfamiliar locations. We also observed how depression adversely affected outcomes in chronic disease management.

Armed with this clinical angst, we sought a model to fill these gaps. As a Patient-Centered Medical Home, we understood the nature of care coordination and team care and recognized the need for screening for behavioral health disorders; yet, we had failed at previous attempts at co-location. Our initial attempts to fill these gaps were piecemeal and reactionary. We knew integration was our next step. Integration, however, can mean different things to different people and we needed a specific definition and criteria to follow. We needed a model to encompass the big picture to see the forest and, at the same time, provide an effective and consistent structure to identify the trees.

In preparation for applying to the ACT grant, I discovered Evolving Models of Behavioral Health [4]. This document provided the structure we needed to outline our program and direct our efforts by introducing the concept of four quadrant clinical integration. They clearly defined the terms—coordination, co-location, and integration—and from the continuum of coordination to integration proposed eight models of care depending on your capacity, resources, and goals. Similar to the NCQA PCMH, this document gave us the blueprint, guidance, and infrastructure we needed to develop our model of care.

Although unaware of this transformation tool, we mirrored the GROW Pathway [5] to integrate our model—Goal setting, Resource assessment, Options, and Work development. Well into our integration process, we discovered another document that helped refine our approach and validate our direction, Organized Evidence-Based Care: Behavioral Health Integration [6]. It would have saved a lot of time and energy if we had access to these documents at the beginning of our journey. These documents categorized and organized the major issues to address in transformation and provided a stepwise framework to get started.

We chose Solution-Focused Brief Therapy (SFBT) as the primary treatment model for our practice. SBFT focuses on problem-solving current issues and takes a goal-oriented approach that helps the patient move toward a desired future while exploring how their solutions involve other people in their life. This model best fit with the dynamics, time resources, and workflow of our practice. We wanted to engage our patients with practical and immediate steps to improve their lives and build up from these small "wins" to achieve long-term objectives. SFBT was particularly useful in working with patients with chronic diseases by focusing on patient strengths and resources.

Financial Planning Focuses on Nonrevenue Gains

The future is already here – it's just not evenly distributed.
William Gibson

CB Many of you might be looking at this section first to determine how to afford behavioral health integration. As noted in the Introduction, there is a "tension of opposites" to offer behavioral health services and to financially afford it (or actually see a positive net income). If you are hoping to read an erudite business plan on

TABLE 4.2 Tips, questions, and considerations for financial planning

Tasks to complete	Tips, questions, and considerations
Determine your financial plan for clinical operations	• In your plan, be cautious not to improve quality at the expense of your financial stability • Does your state or the health plans covering your patients prohibit billing for both medical and behavioral health services on the same day? • What alternative means of financing BHC services are available (codes specific to integrated care, alternative payment models)? • If using an external partner, what health plans are accepted by the BHC partner? The BHC should accept at least 80% of the practice's health plans • Explore and negotiate a "1st free" consultation with the BHC to reduce the patient's financial/emotional barriers. The duration of this introductory visit may be shortened so as not to limit your BHC's visit access and capacity

TABLE 4.2 (continued)

Tasks to complete	Tips, questions, and considerations
Determine your up-front financial "risk-tolerance" and budget for 3 years of integration	• How much money can you spend in up-front investment or costs to start integration without jeopardizing your practice's financial health? Work with your certified public accountant • Forecast a projected 3-year profit-loss statement and balance sheet; run the Quick Acid Test (goal ≥1) and Total Debt to Total Assets (goal <0.50) to expose the potential of becoming insolvent • In the profit-loss statement, include up-front costs for a BHC such as equipment, computers, desk, supplies, software or EHR provider license, capital improvements, rent, medical provider/staff nonrevenue generating time, and costs toward integration. Ongoing costs include EHR provider license, rent, continuing medical education, medical provider/staff nonrevenue generating time, and costs toward integration • Estimate the visit productivity necessary to maintain total ongoing costs of a BHC to ensure sustainability in all 3 years of the profit-loss period
Determine "fair market value" for space in your practice, transaction amount, and frequency. Confirm with your legal team	Specific to external partnerships, this may depend on "innovation philosophies" or grant opportunities and expensing requirements
Determine how to reward your providers and staff	This depends on your organization's infrastructure, business, and payment model. Consider offering continuing education to support the new innovation, share stories, and celebrate small wins along the way

how to offer behavioral health integration to generate profits, unfortunately, there is not a business case to argue that behavioral health integration increases revenue for a small, private practice. (Read that last sentence ... again.) While integrated care codes and programs are increasingly available to buffer the losses, in all behavioral health integration efforts, noneconomic gains support the goals of the Quadruple Aim [7]: improving quality of care, improving patient experience, decreasing healthcare costs, and increasing provider and staff well-being. Since these noneconomic gains indirectly influence economic gains, do not underestimate the impact of these noneconomic gains on the overall financial health of your organization. The cultural shift resulting from these noneconomic gains supports successful integration efforts.

Noneconomic gains in behavioral health integration include:

- More meaningful experience among medical and behavioral health clinicians and personal fulfillment by offering collaborative, accessible care to patients. Clinicians enjoy more efficient workflow through timely access to behavioral health.
- Stronger practice culture and staff who want to be engaged as part of solutions resulting in less burnout and lower turnover of team members.
- Enhanced reputation for whole-person, community-based care that attracts new patients. We experienced increased new patient visits specifically because behavioral health services were available. Consider how to best promote your relationship (more on this topic in section "Staff Development and Patient Engagement").
- Increased patient satisfaction with patient-convenient hours and scheduling options. Options support higher volume and reimbursement. Early morning and evening hours are typically high demand (more on this topic in section "Workflows and Clinical Outcomes").

To address costs and profits (or at least enough revenue to start up and continue integration), studies support that behavioral health integration reduces healthcare costs and increases quality of care. One study showed cost savings of $3363 per patient after 4 years of integration [8]. That breaks down to $70 per patient per month (PMPM) healthcare system savings with behavioral health integration. For our small, primary care clinic serving 6000 patients, our upstart costs were approximately $55,000 with ongoing maintenance costs of $51 PMPM.

Broken down further,
$55,000/5 months = $11,000 per month upstart costs
→ $11,000/6000 patients = $1.83 PMPM upstart costs

$1.83 PMPM upstart costs + $51 PMPM ongoing costs
= $53 PMPM to start, implement, and sustain behavioral health into our clinic for 5 months.

Our start-up costs (mostly in-kind services and not cash expenses) included medical director hours researching clinical care models; meeting time preparing for integration activities such as generalized screening; finalizing appropriate paperwork such as integration disclosure and consents to treat; designing promotional materials; and meetings with our Community Mental Health Center partner. As seen in the Gantt chart and each section in this chapter, many of the upstart costs relate to preparing for the implementation phase. Over time with more lessons learned, tools, and resources available from successful integration projects, upstart costs should be lowered to some extent.

The figures above are estimates but point out that cost savings to the healthcare system may be greater than expenses even in a small, primary care clinic. The research from Advancing Care Together was much more robust and sound. One of the best articles available to date is *Start-Up and Ongoing Practice Expenses of Behavioral Health and Primary Care Integration Interventions in Advancing Care Together (ACT) Program* [9]. The article shows promise that behavioral health integration is affordable and such cost information along with evidence on savings could be leveraged with payers. For more on leveraging your business case with payers, see Chap. 8.

There are several ways to fund integration. It is possible to employ your own BHC and follow a traditional fee-for-service model. This model, however, requires substantial investment, grant revenue, or use of coding practices to support (but not entirely pay for) behavioral health integration. There are now various fee-for-service codes such as Health & Behavior codes and codes for case managers and psychiatric review of cases in the Collaborative Care Model that can be used to support costs.

Value-based care payments or shared-savings models in an Accountable Care Organization may allow for more financial flexibility in redistributing revenue toward integration. It is possible that a large or corporate-based practice may have the administrative resources and the ability to negotiate with health plans to optimize contracts to financially support integration. Depending on your location, insurers may be willing to pay a capitated fee for your behavioral health integration efforts. In this case, be sure to have the data to support the implementation and maintenance costs of your program.

The most promising method of funding integration for our clinic was to partner with a Community Mental Health Center that has experience in behavioral health integration and contracts with most health plans. The Community Mental Health Center has more financial flexibility to support primary care. The financial planning can be led or shared by the Community Mental Health Center based on their transparency, resources, and needs. The Vice President of Corporate Business Development at Jefferson Center for Mental Health notes, "the Community Center recognizes the value propositions of a primary care clinic: a guaranteed referral pattern to a BHC."

In our model, the Community Mental Health Center financially funds the total costs for a BHC (salary, benefits, malpractice, licensure). BHC personnel costs total $60–$100 k depending on region and credentials. The primary care clinic must, therefore, focus on maintaining a referral pattern to cover the costs of a BHC. The following productivity breakdown is feasible:

$100,000 annual expenses for a BHC
Divide by the average reimbursement for a typical BHC visit (depends upon contracts, payers, and region).
→ $85/visit
= 1176 visits/year needed to break even for funding a BHC.
Divide by 12 months in the year.
→ 98 patients/month to break even for funding a BHC.
Divide by the average number of BHC work days per month (or convert the number of hours into "days"). At WMC, the average number of working days is 21 days.
→ 4–5 patients/day need to be seen by a full-time (1 FTE) BHC to break even (with 45–60-min visit durations with dedicated administration time).

Based on the patient needs assessment already completed, will the clinical needs fill the BHC capacity? What is the typical referral "attrition" rate in your clinic?

Even though medical providers refer patients and the BHC has access, patients may not complete a scheduled visit. Even with the best promotion strategies, there are "no shows" and cancelations. As integration evolves, however, the rate improves. Review and calculate a rate of missed appointments as a starting place. This rate will be lower than the rate for behavioral health appointments, but a baseline is helpful in assessing progress. Initially, in our clinic, 50% of patients:

(a) Did not visit with the BHC even when scheduled by the BHC
(b) If the patient scheduled, missed the first appointment

Therefore, using the above example, our medical providers initially needed to generate ten referrals per day until our BHC grew a large enough panel to reach schedule capacity. At WMC, serving 6000 patients, our clinical needs fit this approximate breakdown. WMC has enough patients with specific diagnosis or co-morbidities to fund 1.5 FTE BHCs. Naturally, another approach was needed to improve the rate of completed visits. Warm handoffs will be discussed in section "Staff Development and Patient Engagement".

What if the patient needs assessment shows that the primary care practice can only fund 0.5 FTE BHC? The full benefit of behavioral health integration may not be realized; however, it does not mean you should not proceed. With Standing Orders, referral parameters as guidelines, and a consistent plan for medical provider adoption, the providers, staff, and patients can fund a BHC. See more on this topic in section "Workflows and Clinical Outcomes". Sharing a BHC with another practice is another consideration.

To make the partnership work, a primary care practice can share expenses with a Community Mental Health Center. Offer clinic space, EHR access, and supplies for integration in-kind to the Community Mental Health Center. The BHC needs a "home" or dedicated space for patient visits. With consolidation of policies and protocols and digital promotion, discussed in the subsequent sections, the supplies needed for the BHC do not substantially add to operational expenses and can be absorbed by the practice. EHR access is not an additional expense as the vendors allow for "resources" rather than provider "licenses" that result in zero cost. These in-kind expenses are minimal to a primary care practice and appreciated by a Community Mental Health Center.

There are expenses that did change the clinic financial health. Project how behavioral health integration may shift the company's financials.

Economic gains or increased revenue occur as a result of:

- Increased medical visits because behavioral health issues were identified more consistently through screening and standing orders
- Increased patient visits as a result of community awareness

Economic losses or decreased revenue occur as a result of:

- Co-management of patient care with a BHC.
- Care team meeting time.
- Extended time in check-in to rooming workflow (longer patient visits lead to fewer patient visits).
- Offering in-kind space for a BHC increased rent as a non-revenue generating space.
- Clinicians and staff may expect wage increases with continuous transformation efforts that result in expansion and complexity of their clinical duties.

Robust workforce salary data do not exist for primary care staff who have expanded their job description and integrated behavioral health into their workflow. It is a major challenge to build a team and culture when compensation does not match efforts and performance. The morale of clinicians and staff is impacted when the consistent message is: you are offering care that cannot be found in many places; you are saving lives but we cannot increase your pay.

To improve morale, form a wellness strategy to support performance and productivity. Johnson & Johnson reported from 2002 to 2008, for every dollar spent on employee wellness, the return on investment was $2.71 [10]. Another study suggests an organization with happy employees is 12% more productive [11]. Maintaining a positive culture cannot be done *for* staff but can be done *with* staff. In general, an organization can provide all-staff team building and coaching. Consider offering training on an Optimal Healing Environment [12] or by convening a clinic-employer wellness committee. Alternatively, staff engagement surveys such as the Gallup12 or The Mini Z Burnout Survey offer insight to start addressing culture. Some individuals are "fatigued" for short periods of time and only need small inspirations and positive reinforcement. This is not a strategy to retain all employees because an evolving culture naturally leads to either a change in staff or change in oneself.

WMC improved our staff performance and efficacy in several ways. Staff listened to a series of self-reflection activities and personal goal-setting inspirational talks. Middle-management positions established new personal and professional performance goals two to three times a year. Our Health Coach offered free consultations to staff and conducted numerous group wellness activities. Cultural improvements had a small, although debatable, return on investment through improved productivity and staff retention. The capacity for our clinic to reach our goals, however, was only possible through emphasis on cultural development as the foundation of integration efforts.

Although the *right* staff remain at an organization for meaningfulness and purpose [13], a primary care clinic cannot expect to facilitate employee growth or retain strong staff and providers without paying wages equal or slightly higher to the marketplace. To reward integration accomplishments, slowly increase wages (an economic loss or increased expense) and consider an "all-for-one, one-for-all" approach in profit sharing. Profit sharing is the most tangible, rewarding measure of success for staff. When profit sharing, use both objective and subjective measures and define a formula to fit your company such as team-ness, clinical or operational performance, and contributions to comprehensive services. To more "evenly distribute" the reward for "being the future—now," share profits with all staff and providers. Alternatively, increasing benefits may work best in your organization. You can incentivize your staff with flexible work schedules, non-clinical opportunities for research, teaching or supervision, as well as additional paid time-off.

RSH Fifty-four percent of primary care physicians report burnout, and this percentage seems to be rising yearly [14]. To maintain motivation, we used Daniel Pink's triad—Autonomy, Mastery, and Purpose—to refuel our clinicians and staff with the positive energy needed to implement change by promoting self-direction, by providing the skills and resources to be successful, and by nurturing their personal meaning in work [15]. BHCs can also feel isolated if they are the only BHC in a practice, which may contribute to burnout; helping BHCs connect to a network of other BHCs for professional development and support can provide a buffer against this isolation.

Victor Frankl said, "When we are no longer able to change a situation, we are challenged to change ourselves." Our patients cannot wait for payment reform. Grant funds are difficult to obtain and are short-term solutions. Loans are costly. Although it is difficult to do the "right thing" while balancing competing needs and interests, we chose to maintain our innovations through salary reductions for owners, wage freezes, and temporarily increasing work hours. We are fortunate that all of our clinicians are personally invested in our patients and willing to take ethical action and sacrifice for this professional and social responsibility. This sacrifice, however, was more related to the implementation and maintenance of the Patient-Centered Medical Home than it was for integrating behavioral health. Our current model of "partnering" with the Community Mental Health Center is viable and sustainable once you have spent the time and effort to create an effective infrastructure and strong care teams.

BHC Recruitment and Partnership

> You cannot dream yourself into a character; you must hammer and forge yourself one.
> Henry David Thoreau

CB Integrating a BHC did not happen just once. WMC had been working on integration for 25 years and we have employed or co-located eight BHCs over this time. BHCs left the practice for various reasons. One had a love for children and school-based programs. Another had experience with crisis in the emergency department and was unable to adapt to an outpatient model of care. One had experience and willingness to work in primary care, but determined her passion was in maternal mental health and transitioned to a federally qualified health center.

After three BHCs over 3 years of the ACT grant, it was clear WMC needed to work more closely with the Community Mental Health Center because our needs were not being met. (Many of the principles described here also apply to internal BHC hiring. For additional tips on hiring a BHC internally, see Chap. 6). This was an opportunity for WMC to rethink our needs and develop new criteria for success: skill set, passion, and cultural synergy. I had not developed a BHC job description until this time. Managerially speaking, we had a

Table 4.3 Tips, questions, and considerations for establishing your BHC partnership

Tasks to complete	Tips, questions, and considerations
Discuss sharing leadership and supervision with the Community Mental Health Center	• Explore and determine your role in BHC interviewing and hiring. Use a guideline for interviewing and hiring a BHC that meets both yours and their needs. See Chap. 6 for additional tips • Explore co-supervisory expectations for a BHC. Why, what, and how will you and a partner co-supervise?
Draft a BHC job description	• Embrace your BHC as "one of you" to be adopted into your team. Match the job description to the patient population needs assessment, model of therapy, ideal credentials or experience, and staff-provider culture building assets • Review the Eight Competencies for BHCs [16] for a broader view of the role (See Appendix B)

general idea of BHC skill sets needed at WMC, but the Community Mental Health Center was the hiring organization. Was it my place to share WMC expectations with the hiring personnel at the Community Mental Health Center? We did not want to overstep our role, seem ungrateful, or undermine the hiring protocol. The short answer, however, was yes, and it was a crucial step toward shared leadership.

The practice manager or administration team must participate in the hiring process alongside the Community Mental Health Center. This critical step will facilitate finding the right fit from the start. Prior to a meeting, ask the medical providers to share the BHC skills sets and characteristics they believe result in the best collaboration. Determine the medical providers' personalities, practice styles, strengths, obstacles, and defining descriptors of a collaborative environment. Armed with this information, you can develop a general concept of a BHC who would best fit in your setting. Then, schedule a meeting with the Community Mental Health

Center to share the Community Needs Assessment and to define the "best hire" to meet the primary care expectations. In this meeting, discuss how behaviors and actions, communication styles, and passion translate into cultural synergy that leads to primary care collaboration.

In a job description, how does this translate into personal BHC traits that ensure collaborative care?

When WMC interviewed BHCs, the physical space was described and viewed in order to gauge their desire and willingness to work in the environment. This type of environment is not suited for every individual (regardless of medical or behavioral credentials or position within a clinic). This concept is easily overlooked and can make or break integration at the clinic.

Not surprisingly, patients have a preference for what they need for an optimal BHC experience. Patients want a BHC with strong listening skills, the ability to develop actionable steps, personality characteristics that instill trust, and follow-up that demonstrates personalized care rather than "being just another patient."

Beyond personal characteristics, what credentials and licensure are most appropriate for your care model?

The Community Mental Health Center and primary care providers discussed the differences in credentials and defined a group of individuals best suited for our integration site. In addition, there are rich resources available to help identify the competencies to best deliver integrated care. The Vice President of Corporate Business and Development at Jefferson Center for Mental Health says to hire the best clinicians, not "integration experts" [17].

WMC created a job description in accordance with our primary care needs, role, and responsibilities. After drafting an integrated version, I sent the new job description to the Community Mental Health Center to guide the recruitment process. Although the Community Mental Health Center was bound by regulations to use their own job description, their response was positive. They agreed for WMC to conduct second interviews for strong candidates. I used our job description as a guide to ensure our expectations were met.

We needed to find a BHC to stand the test of time to show integration was sustainable. Outlining the position in a detailed job description proved the key to finding the right person.

When hiring a BHC, ask:

1. What are your clinical passions?
2. Describe the organization and people you ideally want to work with and for.
3. Please share a couple of examples of innovation and creativity. What has been your project management experience?
4. Please share your experience and role at a clinic with integrated behavioral health. What was successful and what can we improve upon here?
5. Please describe the type of environment in which you work best related to physical space, interruptions, and fast-paced cultures.
6. How would you characterize your style of communication with patients? With providers? With staff? Please share examples.
7. What is your scope of care?
8. What do patients misunderstand about you? What do staff and providers misunderstand about you?

Once hired, onboarding the new BHC occurs over 2–4 weeks. The BHC should initially begin onboarding at the Community Mental Health Center and then proceed with the practice introduction. The goal of the onboarding process is to educate the BHC on the practice's operations and build an initial rapport. The BHC should spend time in each department of the primary care practice: understanding scheduling with the front office, experiencing team care by shadowing medical assistants and providers, discovering responsibilities of the care coordinator, and learning about operations from the administration-billing team. The onboarding process also includes spending time with the extended care team: certified health coach (nutrition, exercise, and self-management), chiropractor (physical health services and dry needling), and the care manager (advanced care planning, social needs resources, and tasks based on patient risk stratification per clinic protocols) to provide a complete picture of operations and services. There are other methods for successfully onboarding behavioral health professionals worth exploring [18].

In conjunction with hiring a new BHC, internal job descriptions for staff and medical providers need updating based on new or revised policies, protocols, and workflows, as well as to incorporate the Community Mental Health Center's BHC processes. Beyond supplies and materials discussed as in-kind expenses, your staff resources are also shared by the nature of integration.

RSH It is rewarding and a privilege to work with such caring people in an atmosphere of hope; and when you have the right team, it is like breathing the same breath. It takes a special BHC to merge with primary care. They must have the courage to face both the uncertainty of uncharted territory and the fortitude to meet the distressing challenges of stretching their personal boundaries. This pioneer spirit to find a better way and to make a better place takes an open-minded, resilient, and positive person. A sense of humor helps, but it is mostly about willingness to change. Not every BHC has these characteristics to join such a journey. Over time, we developed a sense with whom we wanted to hold hands, and, similar to starting any relationship, it is a feeling. In an interview, if you can feel excitement and enthusiasm from the BHC candidate as you describe your model, you may have found your teammate. Given this foundation of the compatible characteristics, it is easy to provide the tools to build collaborative skills needed to create an integrative model.

Our physicians and mid-levels are co-located in the same room. We believe this provides improved access to the team leader, improves coordination of care, and adds to the cohesiveness of the team. Our most successful strategy for integrating the BHC was to initially have her join us in this space. She learned our customs, mores, responsibilities, frustrations, and workflow and developed an intimate understanding of primary care. Although close-working environments slowed their visit-to-visit time, clinicians agreed that the opportunity for interactions is necessary for collaboration. The primary care clinicians built trust and communication with the BHC due to this proximity. Each BHC validated that this was the most critical step for them to become "part of the team." Rose Gunn et al. [19] describe this concept as "bumpability," an occurrence resulting from sharing physical space in which medical providers and BHCs work, to enhance spontaneous contact. By sharing space and using our Compact as a Rosetta Stone, we developed both an emotional and working bond that laid the groundwork to move forward on our journey.

Staff Development and Patient Engagement

Talk does not cook rice.
Ancient Chinese Proverb

To give real service you must add something which cannot be bought or measured with money, and that is sincerity and integrity.
Douglas Adams

CB Although we already developed effective communication through building care teams, there are challenging features unique to behavioral health integration. Patient-staff communication barriers exist. Staff need training on how to approach an angry patient or a patient in crisis. Continuous assessment, coaching, and reassessment are critical in the professional development of your staff. For instance, front-office and scheduling personnel often experience emotionally charged patient encounters. If staff do not have the skills to redirect or diffuse the situation, they will experience significant stress throughout integration from inadequate skills to help a patient in need or a situation in which communication is mismatched, misdirected, or misunderstood.

TABLE 4.4 Tips, questions, and considerations for staff development and patient engagement

Tasks to complete	Tips, questions, and considerations
Start with a BH Integration introductory meeting with clinicians Follow with an all-staff meeting to introduce the concept and gather initial feedback	• Introducing a large concept (and change) to staff is typically received well if the medical clinicians are supportive and believe in the idea. Consider asking clinicians to share reasons why integration will benefit patients, clinicians, and staff • All staff will immediately react: "how does this change/benefit my day?"
Develop a tentative 12-month meeting schedule with agenda topics (clinical and administrative)	Schedule process-workflow brainstorming and quality improvement meetings. Ensure all members of the care team, levels of administration, and quality improvement representatives attend
Build in formal patient case discussions in care management meetings and informal discussions during daily huddles (clinical only)	For these meetings to be successful, train all care team members on how to present a patient case using a template to organize their thoughts. Specifically gather feedback from all care team members to make meetings meaningful and actionable
Assess clinician educational needs, areas of interest, and clinical gaps	Educational topics requested by our clinicians: transitioning care from "cure" to "function" in pain management; adverse childhood events; treatment-resistant depression; personality disorders

TABLE 4.4 (continued)

Tasks to complete	Tips, questions, and considerations
Conduct all-staff training	• Training needed for staff in primary care clinics includes: Mental Health First Aid to train staff to de-escalate a situation to get the care the patient needs; customer and compassionate service training; educational series on clinical diagnoses in behavioral health; motivational interviewing; cultural awareness, sensitivity and competency; etiquette for discussing patient care • Train staff to achieve greater self-confidence in caring for patients • Consider the possibility that staff are experiencing their own behavioral health issues. As staff learn about behavioral health diagnoses, they may self-reflect or identify with patients. This highlights a high need for awareness and strong cultural management
Design a promotion strategy for new clinical services	• Include preparing clinicians and staff with messaging, information about the BHC, what patients can expect in a visit with a BHC (in comparison to historical models of behavioral health) • Prior to developing messaging, determine the patient-identified cultures in the population you serve. Consider cultural responsiveness training (cultural competency) and speak to leaders of respective cultures and/or with patients about perceived behavioral health stigma across cultures in your region. Approaching patient communication with awareness of values and beliefs strengthens promotion and well-received messaging

(continued)

TABLE 4.4 (continued)

Tasks to complete	Tips, questions, and considerations
Design an outreach strategy for new clinical services	• Create supporting materials for both staff and patients including a photo and biography of the BHC to compliment a warm handoff or referral to the BHC • Consider sending out a secured portal message to all patients or targeted sub-populations of patients based on updated policies or standing orders • Offer materials in your patient rooms or lobby and update your website and social media
Design a patient survey; design an all-staff and clinician survey	Conduct an initial patient satisfaction survey after 3–6 months of integration implementation. Consider continuing an annual patient satisfaction survey or per-visit patient experience survey

Two training topics are most relevant for behavioral health integration: Mental Health First Aid and compassionate action-customer service. Mental Health First Aid discusses clinical diagnoses, as well as how to approach high-stress, high-need situations. Find specific trainings in your area if you are unable to provide the training yourself. Training should be offered at the beginning of integration implementation followed by a refresher every 1–2 years. Newly hired individuals need training during onboarding. Consider both trainings as an all-staff series. For WMC, the Community Mental Health Center offered Mental Health First Aid training for all Center employees and to the public at no cost.

The second training, compassionate action-customer service, is a series of sessions on general customer service, listening skills, and asking appropriate questions and responding with solutions. As a staff member, "taking compassionate action" in addressing patient concerns is a method of approaching patient situations in a specific frame of mind that focuses on helping those who are suffering. Additional training includes motivational interviewing, framing comments and questions differently, and redefining the purpose of service itself. Advanced topics on sensitivity and cultural competency should be embedded into the overall curriculum. These trainings address verbal and written communication barriers with patients.

To further engage patients, materials need to be developed for patient workflows and for any online promotions. Numerous resources are available from the Agency for Healthcare Research and Quality (AHRQ) Academy for Integrating Behavioral Health and Primary Care and the AIMS Center at the University of Washington [20, 21]. In the clinical setting, the best method of introducing the BHC to patients is face-to-face warm handoffs in which the clinician directly introduces the patient to the BHC. Warm handoffs establish trust and decrease the fears and uncertainty that are barriers to care for patients (and clinicians, at least at first). For a suggested approach to warm handoffs, see Chap. 6.

Patients appreciate a flier that introduces the BHC with their biography, interests, and photograph. The flier increases the patient's perception that the BHC is friendly, open minded, and approachable, as well as answers questions on what type of care is offered and what to expect. Finally, state pertinent statistics or public health messages on the flier to share with patients that they are not alone in their condition.

WMC noted that patients missed appointments more frequently if referred or virtually introduced via the flier as opposed to personal, warm handoffs. WMC also attempted phone call handoffs. Even this method of outreach to patients by the BHC was not as effective as a face-to-face interaction. In the WMC experience, after 12–18 months of integration, patients no longer cautiously approached seeing the BHC; clinicians referred patients regularly; and visits are filled on a consistent basis using a combination of warm handoffs and fliers.

RSH If being out on a limb is a good thing because that is where the fruit is, then, primary care suffers from a high glycemic load. Although trained in behavioral health diagnosis and treatment, our scope of care is limited by our individual experience and interest and, frequently, we are stretched beyond our skill set in diagnosis, treatment, and pharmaceutical management due to the many barriers previously discussed.

Part of our model was to create educational support, both inside and outside the practice, to raise the competencies and confidence of our primary care team.

Medical providers led monthly all-team care management meetings that followed a WMC-designed format—PEP—Policy, Education, and Patient Care. Extended care team providers and cross-departmental staff are included at these meetings. Each person is expected to participate and share ideas or aspects of the whole patient that may or may not be known to the others. Many times, front-office personnel or medical assistants are aware of social and personal information germane to the care plan. Challenging cases are explored, and the dialogue generated between members—medical assistant to health coach to provider to BHC—is robust and enlightening.

Our Community Mental Health Center offered a series of talks every 2 months targeted to our clinicians' interests and needs such as personality disorders, adverse childhood experiences, and treatment-resistant depression. These sessions are a favorite meeting for our providers and have clearly boosted the quality of care we deliver.

Whether you call it a pre-consultation exchange or a psychiatry curb-side consult, access to specialty psychiatry services is a glaring need in primary care. Through our partnership, we arranged for urgent or emergent phone consultation within 24 hours with a psychiatrist at the Community Mental Health Center. Although not used often, it is a joyful experience to have the support. If your organization has the capacity, this can also be accomplished by regular, monthly or biweekly, care management meetings with the psychiatrist for challenging cases; this is a component of the Collaborative Care Model and TEAMCare.

Workflows and Clinical Outcomes

> Obstacles are those frightful things you see when you take your eyes off the goal.
>
> Henry Ford

RSH T.S. Eliot said, "Human kind cannot bear very much reality" and, indeed, clinicians are overwhelmed with excessive decision-making. Many years ago, Mark Ebell M.D., M.S., reported at a conference that family medicine residents made 960 decisions per week or 8 decisions per patient. Undoubtedly, this number has markedly increased with the complexity of practice. One cannot win this battle, but you can mitigate the burden by choosing measures wisely, eliminating wasteful EHR work, developing standing orders, sharing prevention and screening with staff, and by providing medical resources at the point of care.

Developing policies and processes alongside changing culture is like asking someone to start walking on his or her hands. The world turns upside down by challenging your belief system, questioning your knowledge base, and threatening your professional role. Eric Hoffer, American philosopher, succinctly states, "every new adjustment is a crisis in self-esteem." There are already many moving parts to delivering primary care without the addition of innovation projects. We needed the right tools to complete this work. Some tools we had to discover, some we had to create, and others we already used well.

A critical mistake, and one that I wish I had recognized and addressed earlier, was not fully understanding the nature of teams and their role in successfully implementing new workflows. There is a continuum of teams from parallel to consulting to coordinating to multidisciplinary to collaborative [22]. Parallel teams operate as internal silos; for example, with three clinicians, you have four ways of doing things. This creates chaotic and dangerous workflows. We undertook the long process of standardizing clinical documentation and developing templates and protocols to unify our practice and implement high reliable, accountable, and consistent workflows accepted by all of our clinicians.

Everyone must take personal ownership in making change and this only occurs when the clinician or staff recognizes the problem, acknowledges their part in it, and sees himself or herself as part of the solution. In general, this is an attitude

TABLE 4.5 Tips, questions, and considerations for workflows and clinical outcomes

Tasks to complete	Tips, questions, and considerations
Introduce the Collaborative Guidelines and commit to a partner and BHC	• Review the Collaborative Guidelines aka Compact with the leadership, management, and BHC from the Community Mental Health Center • Determine what elements of the four domains are possible "now" and create a plan to satisfy others in the future • Consider using the framework called *The 5A's* to engage your partner in becoming a Behavioral Health Medical Neighbor

Develop policies and standing orders (clinical and administrative)	• Consider your BHC as a specialist rather than a "dumping ground" for any and all behavioral health conditions.
	• The goal is not to "dump" patients onto a BHC but work together in a co-management relationship (see Compact in Appendix A)
	• Policies and standing orders needed for a primary care clinic:
	  (*Administrative*) – Notice of Privacy Practices for Protected Health Information; Protected Health Information consent to transfer medical records; Compliance policy for privacy and security including annual training; clinic payment policy including addressing missed appointments; access and communication policies for patients; Personal Privacy Policy: the patient declines "integration" and desires privacy with no written or verbal communication between BHC and medical provider
	  (*Administrative and clinical*) – discharge and inactivation; active patient empanelment; consent and treatment of minors
	  (*Clinical*) – Behavioral health screening for all patients (e.g., start with new patients or those with certain co-morbidities such as chronic illness, chronic pain); care management and care coordination policies and protocols including patient risk stratification; standardization and documentation of clinical measures in the EHR

Tasks to complete	Tips, questions, and considerations
Create an implementation timeline	• All policies and standing orders cannot be implemented at once. Choose one to two policies to focus on first; in 3 months, add two more policies; repeat every quarter • Early attention on developing or revising policies and standing orders will provide a starting place for all providers and staff to frame conversations, act in practice, and work together in a tangible way
Develop a workflow	Diagram workflow and write in a checklist format
Develop a chart of clinical quality measures and standardized documentation in the EHR	The columns of the chart should include measure, numerator, denominator, patient population age, staff responsible for documenting in an EHR, very detailed description of location of documentation in EHR. See Chap. 7 for more details on measurement for quality improvement
Develop supporting materials that detail expanded clinical elements of policies, standing orders, and workflows	• Supporting materials needed for a primary care practice to assist evidence-based *clinical decision making*; clinical parameters for automatic referrals vs. shared-decision referrals vs. self-referrals; definitions of high-acuity patients vs. patients with complicated lives; emergent referral vs. routine referral criteria and access expectations • Supporting materials needed for a primary care practice to assist standardized *workflows*: a checklist for pre-visit, visit, and post-visit. Organize the checklists by responsible individuals (front desk staff, medical assistants, providers, BHCs, care manager, care coordinator, billing personnel) • Consider using a bubble-diagram format instead of checklists depending on staff learning styles

rather than a skill set. Our approach was to study team building and implement effective strategies for team meetings. Initially, we scheduled weekly, hour-long team meetings in which we built bidirectional communication and trust; discussed and established roles for improving accountability and communication; assessed our dysfunctions as a team [23]; and reviewed forming, storming, norming, and performing concepts [24]. Most importantly, we set and committed to the goals as a group [25] using AIM Statements. Only then were we able to successfully initiate and implement new workflows.

The simple task of screening our core measures was not so simple. It took 6 months to identify which measures to track, create a process to determine who was responsible to obtain and record the measure, what specific language to use, and in exactly what field to report it in the EHR. The process, of course, had to ensure that this information was available to and actionable by the clinician. When completed, we found our reach (percentage of patients screened) markedly improved. All the clinicians had a different approach to treating behavioral health problems and a different threshold on when to refer. After review of the literature, we chose an algorithm to become our standard and circulated it among the providers. When we were communicating well and following the same protocols, with respect to individual variances, we knew we had progressed to a coordinating team. As we included other team members, we became a multidisciplinary team. Through various meetings and workshops, we learned to share leadership and transformed to a collaborative team.

We were then ready to reach out to behavioral health and integrate a BHC as a collaborative team member. We had to re-form, re-norm, re-storm to perform. Asking others to integrate with us is similar to changing behavior in patients, so we used a model that with which we were familiar, the 5 A's Behavior Change Model—Ask, Advise, Assess, Assist, and Arrange. We discussed the first three A's in Chap. 3.

To Assist in helping the Community Mental Health Center and BHC become part of our team, we created several tools. The Compact, also discussed in Chap. 3, assisted the

Community Mental Health Center and BHC to understand their responsibilities and expectations. To facilitate bidirectional communication in the same EHR, we developed templates for transition of care records utilizing the ADAPT acronym.

We all know the pros and cons of the EHR; however, in integration it is especially important as a conduit for bidirectional information and a platform for a shared care plan. When I see a patient in counseling, it is extremely helpful to be able to see the BHC consultation and support his or her plan when I visit with the patient. Imagine the comfort the patient experiences when I am aware of his or her issues and able to discuss, problem-solve, and support the BHC's treatment plan. From the BHC perspective, they receive the referral with a specific request from the provider with pertinent information about the patient that facilitates her intake process.

Assessment	New/changed primary and secondary diagnoses with ICD 10 codes, controlled versus uncontrolled.
Decision-making	Supportive evidence and logic for diagnosis, differential diagnosis, and rationale for treatment with medication or cognitive therapies.
Advice to patient and patient goals	Summarize information, patient education, and community resources provided to patient. Specify patient goals and methods to activate/engage patient in their care.
Plan	Recommended treatment plan and expectations with timeline of future tests or secondary referrals and who is responsible to institute, coordinate, follow up, and manage the information.
Task List	Outline next steps in treatment and who is responsible for each task; specify when the patient should return to the medical clinician.

Two additional strategies stand out to Assist our BHC. We created two tools that we believe are most important to support collaboration and match demand with BHC capacity.

- Referral Request Policy—A critical issue in transition of care is how to define emergent and routine referrals from the clinician to the BHC. In a single meeting, clinicians and the BHC discussed their needs and concerns and, through open dialogue, an agreement was rapidly reached. These definitions were written into policy and distributed to the entire staff: "emergent"/"urgent" referred patients are to be seen by the BHC within 2–3 calendar days, "routine" within 2–3 calendar weeks.
- Referral Access Tool—Medical providers also needed a real-time communication tool to manage referral "flow" and patient access. This tool established a priority system for referrals to the BHC. The BHC designed a Green-Yellow-Red "traffic" light that was posted in the provider office as a visual representation of BHC availability. A Green light indicated unrestricted access. A Yellow light indicated a lack of appointment slots in the next 2 weeks and thus, clinicians needed to manage the care until an appointment was available. A Red Light meant medical clinicians needed to manage their patients until the BHC changed her status. During Yellow and Red light status, medical clinicians still had access to the BHC for urgent or emergent advice but referrals were determined on an individual basis after a "curb-side" consult. Warm handoffs for crisis intervention are always available.

The Community Mental Health Center and the BHC, in turn, assisted us through educational programs and constructive feedback to increase our knowledge base and treatment skills, expanding our scope in delivering behavioral healthcare and decreasing the demand for BHC referral.

To Arrange, we held monthly meetings to continue problem-solving and ensure our plan stayed on track as discussed in section "Staff Development and Patient Engagement".

Many of our tools, screening policies, and standing orders were created in the process of becoming a PCMH. Fortunately, a general policy or workflow can serve as a template for future policies and protocols, easing your workload. Our process of creating a workflow or standing order became standardized as follows:

1. Identify a need.
2. Perform a literature search to find, if available, a comprehensive review or white paper that outlines the details to be addressed.
3. Determine your goal, considering your needs and resources.
4. Filter and fit the elements into the most suitable policy or procedure template.
5. Obtain feedback from staff.
6. Pilot with a small team.
7. Implement into the practice.

Voila, you are done.

There are always exceptions that confound protocols or skirt policies. Patients will sometimes self-refer to our BHC and request that information is not shared with the clinician. Other patients seek behavioral healthcare from therapists outside our office from whom we rarely receive communication. Although these circumstances perpetuate fragmentation of care, we respect the patient's decision and try to support the care the best we can.

CB The Navy Seals advise that transformation is long and slow. "The 'all-out, all the time' approach is counterproductive. We can never repeat enough importance of taking a long-term approach to training, and to encourage SEAL candidates to focus on achieving consistent, gradual progress over several months, rather than trying to achieve instant gratification and stupendous results right now" [26].

Clinicians and staff must know each team member's role and responsibilities, anticipate behavior and action, foster high reliability and accountability with one another, and reduce expectations for immediate "stupendous results." Full integration of behavioral health is an advanced model and fosters high expectations. Early in the implementation process, address the fears or concerns of not satisfying the expectations of integration work. At times, aspects of integration will evolve in uncertain directions due to organizational needs. A best practice is to share with staff and clinicians that implementing a policy and workflow will be slow, inexact, and not perfect.

WMC defined a tolerance level for "successful" or "acceptable" degrees of implementation consistent with "The 80/20 Rule." There is not a protocol that can account for all patient scenarios, even practicing evidence-based, safe, personalized medicine. Eighty percent of the time, the policy is relevant or the process will work; 20% of the time, the policy is not appropriate or the process will not work for operational or patient-centered reasons. In meetings, staff used the 80/20 Rule to discuss policy and workflow to easily move past the seemingly impossible barriers to implementation for every patient scenario.

Although we used the 80/20 Rule, advancing behavioral services over time led to more complexity and challenges. It is especially important to find solutions for the outlying 20% as these situations cause the most stress and work for staff and clinicians. Define a plan for how to make decisions or change workflow for the 20% that require a workaround to correct an imperfect policy. The manager should determine operational next steps when staff experience such an exception. Ask the physician champion for advice when the situation involves clinical care. Staff want to "do a good job" and resolve problems for the sake of the patient and their care. Over time, clinicians and staff learned how to provide solutions without additional oversight or support.

Consider offering a venue for discussing small details. It is highly recommended to gather feedback from all positions in a clinic. Unknowingly, it is easy to miss a perspective that may change a workflow. Build a culture in which positions are level and voices heard. The goal of meetings is to allow enough time for finding the small issues that may occur within the bigger workflow and agree upon a plan to minimize the issue before it becomes a larger one.

WMC historically spent an entire hour drafting an initial workflow to implement a policy or standing order. Everyone's perspective was needed to create a better, more efficient, and adoptable workflow. As a result of building effective and inclusive team meetings, after the first 12–18 months of integration, conversations regarding workflow decreased to 30 min and later 15 min per meeting.

Once an initial workflow is accepted, pilot the new protocol with a small team. Once clinicians and staff are comfortable following a new workflow and reviewing data regularly, a phenomenon occurs in which they raise their personal expectations and desire to implement a process closer to perfection.

After a consistent policy is implemented with a standardized, reliable, nearly perfect workflow, the volume of protocols, documentation, and data mining increases exponentially. A major challenge in managing the volume is clinician and staff documentation "fatigue." To minimize this issue, a best management practice is to review what data are required across all innovations and health plan clinical quality measures, as well as those that are not required. Write out cross-referenced mapping of the measures to ensure policies and workflows are designed with all initiatives in mind. Then, focus on consolidating policies and workflows for the required measures and reduce the unnecessary documentation.

Clinical priorities include efficient workflows to lead to improved health outcomes. One clinical priority is to develop a BHC schedule that allows for best patient access. There are many scheduling and access scenarios. Delivery of care is influenced and shaped by local context, such as organization size, resources, and patient needs [27]. Use the needs assessment and a demand-capacity analysis in conjunction with your preferred model of care such as Solution-Focused Brief Therapy to define an initial schedule. Determining the frequency of warm handoff requests is also necessary. For any partnership, it may take up to 12 months to balance BHC capacity with demand. A workable schedule for matching patient needs with BHC availability includes:

- Five 45-min visits (includes chart documentation time)
- Five 15-min breaks between each scheduled visit
- Two administrative hours to complete Community Mental Health Center requirements and perform care coordination responsibilities

Other models have shorter visit times and more open access; after getting started, you will fine-tune your schedule with experiential learning. Convenient patient access is best achieved by staggering start and end times for the day. Match the medical provider hours with BHC hours to increase hand-off accessibility. Matching hours and building stronger working relationships increase trust between the two disciplines, generate more referrals, and lead to more financial stability sooner.

Finally, begin the day with scheduled appointments to expand care access and ensure estimated BHC productivity. Scheduled appointments are more reliable and predictable than being able to anticipate the need for warm handoffs to fill the same time. If the scheduled appointments are missed or canceled, it is still possible to fill availability by warm handoffs. To determine specific BHC access hours, consider a study to review when most incoming phone calls are generated and provider referrals for behavioral health are scheduled. Generally, our clinic saw the most need for patient care on Mondays, Tuesdays, and Fridays. Therefore, the schedule for the BHC on Fridays allowed warm handoffs to address patients with more urgent matters prior to a weekend.

Mondays, Wednesdays	Scheduled appointments	7a, 8a, 10a, 12p, 2p
	Breaks	745a, 845a, 1045a, 1245p, 245p
	Administrative time	9a, 3p
Tuesdays, Thursdays	Scheduled appointments	9a, 10a, 12p, 1p, 3p, 5p
	Breaks	945a, 1045a, 1245p, 145p, 345p, 545p
	Administrative time	11a, 2p, 4p
Fridays	Scheduled appointments	8a, 9a, 10a, 1p, 3p
	Breaks	845a, 945a, 1045a, 145p, 345p
	Administrative time	11a, 2p, 4p

Workflow continues to develop and improve contributing to the noneconomic gains and revenue, previously discussed in section "Financial Planning Focuses on Nonrevenue Gains".

Organize an Integration Project

Continuous improvement is better than delayed perfection.
Mark Twain

A best practice in project management is to use a logic model that outlines implementation with links to vision and mission. Logic models clearly demonstrate the linkages between concepts, resources, activities, and outcomes. The Pell Institute defines your planned work as consisting of Resources/Inputs and Activities, leading to your intended results of Outputs, Outcomes, and Impact [28].

To get started, try building your own logic model to get clarity on how all of the pieces fit together for successful behavioral health integration. Define the Inputs, Outputs, Outcomes, and Impact before completing Activities.

In the example in Table 4.6, Resource/Inputs are those positions/roles/stakeholders involved in integration. "Patients" are listed first because offering behavioral health integration includes patients as part of a care team. The next group is Clinicians, Staff, Community Mental Health Center, BHC, Health Plans, or any other organization that is involved or impacted by integration. Many of the outcomes or goals for patients are also relevant and important to providers, staff, and community centers.

The Activities are the implementation steps to take. Outline the Activities and add sub-activities or Tasks. Link these implementation steps to the Outputs. Note the Activities in the example below are very similar to the Tasks previously outlined in an attempt to show how integration steps are associated with your vision, mission, and Outcomes.

Measures of success (Outcomes, Impact) are generally the same for all organizations, but the details of Activities will be unique to your behavioral health integration model. The vision

TABLE 4.6 Sample logic model

Resources/inputs	Activities	Outputs	Outcomes	Impacts
Patients, BHC, medical clinicians, care manager, care coordinator, support staff, insurers	1. Implement paper or electronic screening for all patients at check-in 2. Define and discuss referral parameters with medical team, including standing orders 3. Create patient engagement tools, materials, promotion of new services at the clinic 4. Offer a first visit at zero-charge	1. Patients are screened 2. Patients are referred to BHC 3. Patients are aware of services & experience whole-person care 4. Patients access care, minimizing financial barriers	1. Increase # with behavioral health screening by X% 2. Increase # of BHC referrals by X% (includes self-referrals) 3. Increase patient self-efficacy by X% 4. Increase personal goals reached by X% 5. Increase # of patients with depression improved within 6 months of care by X% 6. Increase patient awareness/exposure of whole-person care by X% 7. Increase patient satisfaction of care by X% due to whole-person care	• Expanded whole-person, personalized, safe, accessible care • Greater patient experience • Improved health outcomes

Activities	Outputs	Outcomes	Impacts
1. Host an introductory meeting for framing and sharing vision
2. Offer a behavioral health education series
3. Introduce and review the medical neighborhood Compact; discuss standardized documentation
4. Develop and introduce standing orders
5. Develop a chart of standardized documentation for measures	1. Clinicians and care teams believe work is meaningful
2. Clinicians and care teams are empowered with knowledge
3. Clinicians are getting the appropriate patient information
4. Safe, standard of care services are provided
5. Care teams are clear about how to document clinical quality measures	(All outcomes listed above) &
1. Decrease provider loss of control and increase well-being measures by X%
2. Increase knowledge base of behavioral health topics and confidence in managing care by X%
3. Improve care coordination and bidirectional communication to BHCs by X%
4. Increase # of patients screened, counseled by X%	• All Impacts listed above
• Increased clinician satisfaction and well-being

and mission elements are added under the Impact section. Chap. 7 further discusses evaluating and measuring Outcomes.

Conclusion

To build an infrastructure capable of sustaining behavioral health integration you must design and slowly adapt the clinical operations, policies, and protocols to support change. Financial sustainability is achieved through utilization of community resources and valuing both revenue and nonrevenue priorities. Finding the right BHC to fit in your model and culture is critical to sustainable success. Develop the tools and processes to create an integrated team. Measure your success and prepare to meet future challenges.

> One never notices what has been done;
> One can only see what remains to be done.
>
> Marie Curie

References

1. Bodenheimer T, Laing B. The teamlet model of primary care. Ann Fam Med. 2007;5:457–61.
2. Albom M. Tuesdays with Morrie. New York: Doubleday; 1997.
3. http://www.jimcollins.com/article_topics/articles/the-flywheel-effect.html
4. Collins C, et al. Evolving models of behavioral health. New York: Milbank Memorial Fund; 2010.
5. Ratzliff A, et al. Practical approaches for achieving integrated behavioral health care in primary care settings. Am J Med Qual. 2017;32(2):117–21.
6. Safety Net Medical Home Initiative, Ratzliff A. In: Phillips KE, Holt BS, editors. Organized, evidence-based care supplement: behavioral health integration. Seattle, WA: Qualis Health, MacColl Center for Health Care Innovation at the Group Health Research Institute, and the University of Washington's AIMS Center; 2014.
7. Bodenheimer T, Sinsky C. From triple to quadruple aim: care of the patient requires care of the provider. Ann Fam Med. 2017;12(6):573–6.

8. Unützer J, et al. Long-term cost effects of collaborative care for late-life depression. Am J Manag Care. 2008;14(2):95–100.
9. Wallace NT, et al. Start-up and ongoing practice expenses of behavioral health and primary care integration interventions in the Advancing Care Together (ACT) program. J Am Board Fam Med. 2015;28:S86–97.
10. Berry LL, Mirabito AM, Baun WB. What's the hard return on employee wellness programs? Harv Bus Rev. 2010. https://hbr.org/2010/12/whats-the-hard-return-on-employee-wellness-programs.
11. Oswald AJ, et al. Happiness and productivity. 2015. https://www2.warwick.ac.uk/newsandevents/pressreleases/new_study_shows/.
12. Sakallaris BR, et al. Optimal healing environments. Glob Adv Health Med. 2015;4(3):40–5.
13. Alexander A. The power of purpose: how organizations are making work more meaningful. 2016. http://www.sesp.northwestern.edu/masters-learning-and-organizational-change/knowledge-lens/stories/2016/the-power-of-purpose-how-organizations-are-making-work-more-meaningful.html.
14. Peckham C. Medscape lifestyle report 2016: bias and burnout. Medscape. 2016. http://www.medscape.com/slideshow/lifestyle-2016-overview-6007335.
15. Pink DH. Drive: the surprising truth about what motivates us. New York: Riverhead Books; 2009.
16. Miller BF, Gilchrist EC, Ross KM, Wong SL, Blount A, Peek CJ. Core competencies for behavioral health providers working in primary care. Prepared from the Colorado consensus conference. February 2016.
17. Fishbein D. Developing sustainable behavioral health integration into the PCMH. [Powerpoint slides]. 2016.
18. Hall J, et al. Preparing the workforce for behavioral health and primary care integration. J Am Board Fam Med. 2015;28:S41–51.
19. Gunn R, et al. Designing a clinical space for the delivery of integrated behavioral health and primary care. J Am Board Fam Med. 2015;28:S52–62.
20. Resource Library. AIMS Center. University of Washington. 2018. http://aims.uw.edu/resource-library.
21. Prepare the infrastructure in your setting. The Academy: Integrating Behavioral Health and Primary Care. Agency for Healthcare Research and Quality. https://integrationacademy.ahrq.gov/products/playbook/educate-patients-and-families-about-integrated-ambulatory-care.

22. Boon H, et al. From parallel practice to integrative health care: a conceptual framework. BMC Health Serv Res. 2004;4:15–20.
23. Lencioni P. The five dysfunctions of a team: a leadership fable. San Francisco: Jossey-Bass; 2002.
24. Tuckman BW. Developmental sequence in small groups. Psychol Bull. 1965;63(6):384–99.
25. Cassidy K. Tuckman revisited: proposing a new model of group development for practitioners. J Experiential Educ. 2016;29(3):413–7.
26. Training. Official Naval Special Warfare Website. http://www.sealswcc.com/navy-seal-training.html.
27. Davis MM, et al. Clinician staffing, scheduling, and engagement strategies among primary care practices delivering integrated care. J Am Board Fam Med. 2015;28:S32–40.
28. EvaluationToolkit. Using a logic model. The Pell Institute for the Study of Opportunity in Higher Education. 2018. http://toolkit.pellinstitute.org/evaluation-guide/plan-budget/using-a-logic-model/.

Chapter 5
Everyone Leads

Frank Verloin deGruy III and Parinda Khatri

Preamble

Change is often described as "messy." Yet innovators can exert discipline in managing change, just as they exert discipline in other areas of their practice, for example, having a goal that people can relate to, making manageable starts, monitoring to make course corrections, and learning from missteps while staying connected to what matters to people. Everyone leads—not only designated leaders—taking initiative with agreed-upon goals. Behavioral health integration is more than a technical adjustment to familiar methods—it is practice transformation. Transformation involves adaptive leadership—leading change that is disruptive to familiar habits, roles, who you work with every day, and even what counts as a good job. *CJP*

F. V. deGruyIII (✉)
Department of Family Medicine,
University of Colorado School of Medicine, Aurora, CO, USA
e-mail: frank.degruy@ucdenver.edu

P. Khatri
Cherokee Health Systems, Knoxville, TN, USA

Introduction

Everyone leads. We accept Paul Schmitz's notion of leadership as "an action everyone can take and not a position few hold" (see Schmitz under Additional Reading). Through this lens, we view leadership as a *function* rather than a structured role. Thus, this chapter is written not just for the medical director or the clinic manager or the team leader, but for every person who participates in the care of patients and the operation of the clinic. Observe any high-performing clinic and notice the sheer number of people who take responsibility for the care of patients, the operation of the clinic, and show a drive to do what is best for the organization. Note how many people model the aspirational culture of the organization—this is indeed the "secret sauce" to building an exemplary integrated system. The kind of practice transformation described here requires the active participation of all team members *as leaders—taking initiative to accomplish an agreed-upon goal*. For many, this is a difficult notion to digest and describe, and therefore we will take pains to explain and illustrate how this applies throughout the team.

Not everyone exercises leadership in exactly the same way. Clinical work—and the financial and operational work that supports it—is differentiated into a number of interdependent roles, and the operation of leadership within each is likewise differentiated. A chief executive officer (CEO) of a health system and a care manager will have different leadership roles and responsibilities from those actually rendering care on the ground. We will explain and illustrate these differences, as well as the commonalities across different leadership domains.

We view successful clinics not so much as healthcare production factories that efficiently dispense evidence-based treatments in assembly-line fashion, but instead as adaptive management systems designed to support a state of health and wellness for people, whose health concerns, life circumstances, beliefs, and resources are continuously in flux. Personal care plans change all the time, sometimes in ways that could not be anticipated. The primary care clinic is not so much a machine as an organism, subject to the same laws of self-regulation and homeostasis that govern the internal states of all living things.

This is a book about how to make one radical, utterly transformative change in your clinic—how to integrate behavioral health into the fabric of "ordinary" primary care. In truth, this one change is a continuous series of changes or adjustments: a strategy for change with continuous course corrections. This capacity to continuously adjust under continuously changing circumstances *for the purpose of continuously achieving your goals* is a cardinal feature of successful clinics. In viewing primary care clinics as organisms, we will draw from the concept of adaptive management from the fields of ecology and environmental sciences as an effective and efficient process for systemic change. *Complex adaptive leadership* entails adoption of an iterative, structured decision-making process that is based on continuously monitoring processes and outcomes and rapidly responding to deviations and shortfalls.

Why is leadership so important in integration? Blending behavioral health into primary care requires a *practice transformation*. It is not merely the addition of a specialty mental health program attached to a primary care clinic. The underlying assumptions are thus:

- To have a strong healthcare system, you must have a strong primary care system.
- To have a strong primary care system, you must appropriately address behavioral health concerns.
- The overall driver of integration of behavioral health is the need to support the functions of primary care—to give patients clinical care that addresses most or all of their health concerns in a seamless and collaborative fashion.
- To integrate means to enhance access, expand scope, support coordination, and build continuity of care.

In short, integration changes everything. And at this time of historically low morale among clinicians in traditional primary care settings, it is important to emphasize that transformation to an integrated care system will not only result in improved health and quality of care but will also make practice more rewarding, and yes, it will help restore the joy to practice.

This chapter is written in two sections. The first describes the principles that govern successful leadership in the complex adaptive system that is a primary care clinic. The second section describes the exercise of that leadership—what it looks like in the course of integrating and improving a clinic. There is an enormous literature that supports the development and use of these principles, a selection from which is appended to the end of this chapter as additional readings.

Principles of Complex Adaptive Leadership

Let us look at the key elements of an adaptive system, whether it is an organism or an organization, and see what leadership roles follow from these elements. First is *purpose*. To what end do you exist? What are you trying to be? For an organism, you might say it wishes to *live*, autonomously and freely. The preconditions for this, in terms of physiologic limits or parameters, are constrained and not negotiable. Internal temperature needs to be relatively constant at around 98°. Sodium levels, oxygen saturation, blood pressure, urea levels, and countless other variables must remain relatively constant in the face of an external environment that is continuously changing. The majority of an organism's energy goes to maintaining this homeostatic constancy, invisibly, in the face of continuous external challenges to this invariance. In this sense, life abides if certain features of the internal environment can be held constant. For any organization, its purpose is usually described as its *mission*. The mission of a healthcare system usually involves improving the health of its designated community or population. The key preconditions of a healthcare system, to parallel that of a living organization, are physical space, clinical and support staffing, scheduling, financing, electronic health records, processes for referrals, labs, medication refills, credentialing, and so on. Patients "flow through" a healthcare system—this flow must be maintained despite ever-changing variations in the preconditions. Clinicians call in sick. Staff leave. The heating system breaks. Unscheduled patients walk in. A patient presents in suicidal crisis. The appointment software stops working. Payment for a clinical service is reduced. In order to maintain fixity of purpose in the face of a continuously changing external environment, the clinic team must continuously adjust. Leaders create a context in which these "calculations and recalculations," like a GPS programmed for a target destination, can be made quickly and decisively to stay on course to achieve the purpose of the organization. It is important to note that these recalibrations often, if not always, occur with some level of uncertainty. Incomplete understanding, knowledge, and control of all factors affecting the homeostasis are inherent in any organism or ecological system. Strong leaders acknowledge, even embrace, this uncertainty and foster a framework of good decision-making designed to accommodate the influence of unknown variables in the equation.

Leadership in the context of integration means changing — disrupting, if you will — the homeostasis of the health clinic. The very nature of homeostasis is to seek stabilization and "normalcy." The default to the status quo (e.g., siloed behavioral health, fragmented medical care) is a powerful force that requires an even more powerful counterforce to forge a new homeostatic state. Homeostasis is not an unchanging, constant state. Rather, we view homeostasis as a dynamic equilibrium, in which the system is perpetually changing in order to optimize functioning in the midst of ever-shifting and fluctuating external conditions.

There are two principal mechanisms by which these adjustments to external changes are made. The first is a system of sensors and measurement. An organism is continuously making thousands, even millions, of measurements to assess its internal state. If glucose levels or oxygen saturation or blood pressure rise above or fall below a certain threshold, the organism senses this. This process — measurement of internal state — is absolutely indispensable to the maintenance of function. For a clinic, this might be an overwhelming volume of visits for infections during an influenza epidemic, the presence of clinical depression as a comorbid condition in 15% of patients receiving care for chronic diseases, the loss of funding for children's preventive care, the fact that it is requiring over an hour for patients to complete a normal clinic visit, a shortage of local anesthetic, new patient visits are backed up for 3 months, the quality of diabetes care is below guideline recommendations, no-show rates are at 30% — any measurable feature of the function or outcomes of interest, or of factors that are interfering with the clinic's ability to accomplish its mission. Health systems must identify the outcome domains critical to the achievement of their mission. Access, clinical quality, efficiency of workflow, productivity, and patient satisfaction are common outcome domains that require constant monitoring by all team members for optimal organizational functioning. Moreover, the desired outcome should be delineated and the "limits of normal" set to maintain homeostasis of the system. Blending behavioral health into primary care involves modifying some parameters and adding others. How quickly should behavioral health problems be addressed (e.g., same day, 2 weeks, or 2 months for a new appointment)? At what point does it become unacceptable? What percentage of behavioral health problems should be managed within the primary care system? In sum, when should the system sensors signal a problem that needs to be addressed?

The second principal mechanism is the response to this measurement. What adjustments can the organism or the clinic system make to re-equilibrate and restore full function? An organism may secrete a water-retaining hormone, or a vasopressor, or send leukocytes to the site of an infection. A clinic might add a care manager or a behavioral health consultant to the team to expand behavioral health access, implement an advanced access process to reduce no-show rates, or build in decision-making aids to improve quality of care for a chronic health problem. It is in the area of response that high-performing organizations shine, often because their leaders encourage creative problem-solving, rapid-cycle innovation, and experimental solutions. Examples of solutions that were once "imperfect, out-of-the-box" ideas to address a problem but are now standard approaches to care abound. One such example, telemedicine, emerged as an attempt to improve access to care in remote rural areas well before the technology was well developed. Decades ago, embedding a behavioral health clinician into the primary care setting in one of our clinics was the answer to the lack of space available for a formal therapy office in a small rural town; today this is an accepted standard of care. Leaders know unique responses to distress signals can strengthen the overall system in the long term.

In summary, these are the three cardinal functions within the healthy operation of a primary care clinic system: set your direction (the purpose), measure how you are doing (sensors and measurement), and adjust accordingly (respond to the measurement). In a clinic system, it is the role of leaders to initiate and oversee each of these, and in the sections below we will spell out how each of these looks in practice. In large systems these roles might be served by different people with differentiated leadership responsibilities, but in small clinics these leadership functions might be met by the same person or group of people. Regardless of size, however, the processes and components of integrated systems are complementary and interdependent. Each change, no matter how small, impacts (or better, *disrupts*) a number of parts that make up the whole of the organization. Oversight, guidance, and direction are necessary in this ultra-sensitive machinery of integrated healthcare delivery.

Set a Vision and a Mission for Your Organization

This is your polestar. The leader is the magnet that passes over everyone working there, to point them in the same direction and keep them pulling together for the same thing: something larger than themselves. This vision or mission statement must be simple, memorable, and inspiring. Every action, every decision, every clinical gesture must comport with it. Every member of the organization must be able to say it as a tagline or a mantra and show that whatever they are doing at the moment maps to it. Examples of statements developed by successful integrated clinics are, "We envision all the people in our community receiving comprehensive, integrated whole-person care"; or "We are here to make sure everyone who needs healthcare gets it"; or "We aspire to make this the healthiest county in the state"; or "We will work together to address all of our patients' healthcare needs." Notice that in these examples vision and mission are somewhat commingled. Both are necessary — you need purpose as well as direction — but it is less important that you create clear boundaries between mission and vision than that you craft a statement that says what you are trying to do or why you exist. Writing a mission or vision statement is commonly thought of as an administrative task, but it is not the sole responsibility of administrative leaders (i.e., those at the highest levels of the organization) to craft this statement — indeed, it is best be done by everyone together. It is, however, a responsibility of the administrative leaders to make sure everyone knows it, agrees to it, says it all the time, and lives by it. That is a serious leadership responsibility. Of course, this statement can and should change over the years, but on a day-to-day basis, it is a constant — the unchanging polestar toward which all efforts are made. The clinic should change when it is not meeting its mission or when a change in the environment knocks it off course and requires a corresponding response to get back on track. In the press of practice, we have a tendency to lose sight of our goal. No sooner do we figure out a solution to a problem than we make the solution our standard operating procedure (SOP), and mindlessly adhere to it even when circumstances change again and our SOP no longer pulls us to our polestar. We mistake the map for the territory. It is easy to get lost without leaders pointing to the polestar. We forget that what is important is staying accessible to our patients, not having an elegant scheduling system. A shared vision keeps us looking together in the right direction — reminds us what we aspire to. There are forms of integration that are tight, elegant, efficient, and effective — until something changes. Then, we must remember that we integrate to give good care, not for the sake of integration as an end in itself. Vigilance about the mission is essential to leadership.

Build the Right Team for Integration

Another function of administrative leadership in an adaptive system is to get the right people together on the team. An example of how this works within an organism might be the development of an immune system that, upon detecting invasion by bacteria, responds on multiple fronts by producing different kinds of antibodies, mediators of inflammation, cells that migrate to the site to neutralize and remove the antigen, and so on—an integrated multipronged response. In a clinic, this same multipronged approach applies. The whole point of putting a team together is because it is the *means* by which goals can be met. It is not the goal itself. If a practice decides they exist to help people become healthier, team-based integrated primary care is known to be generally effective at accomplishing this. You hire and train a team that can deal with the demands of ordinary care and that can also respond to unanticipated demands. It is neither possible nor necessary for team members to fit together perfectly and seamlessly, but it is important to hire people who:

- Share the values and priorities of the organization
- Respect differences and can accommodate to different methods and strategies
- Are steadfast and trustworthy
- Work hard and consistently do more than their share of the work
- Are flexible, can improvise, and can work in a variety of settings
- Understand something about how teams work, can see beyond the limits of their own job descriptions, and make good partners
- Communicate well
- Are interested in and have an aptitude for solving problems
- Appreciate persistence and understand the iterative process
- Care about quality, integrity, and honesty
- Have the specific skills the clinic needs

A good administrative leader learns to find and hire such people. All team members participate in this hiring process.

A team will function better if there is a balance, or complementarity, of strengths and functions among its members. Specifically, a visionary without strong implementation skills would be more effective if joined by an implementer who may not be particularly visionary. A team may benefit from the participation of a bridger who can translate ideas into language understood by all. So in assembling a team, it is important to assess the overall complement of strengths and talents.

Perhaps more challenging than getting the right people on the team, but just as crucial, is getting the wrong people off. Few leaders have the luxury of building a team from scratch. Transforming a system requires identifying the people who are in alignment with the desired change and those who are not. The saying "one rotten apple can ruin the barrel" is a useful reminder of the powerful negative impact of even one person on the ability of a system to make and sustain positive changes to meet its mission. It is the hard job of a leader to assess the influence of each person on the team and make the necessary transitions in staffing to facilitate optimal functioning of the system. The importance of this step cannot be overemphasized. The most effective leaders are willing to make the tough and sometimes unpleasant decisions for change needed for an organization to thrive.

Support a Culture for Team-Based Care in a Complex Adaptive System

A culture is comprised of the beliefs, behaviors, opinions, customs, and attitudes that characterize a group of people—in this case a clinic or healthcare system. Most of us acquired a set of cultural norms implicitly, while growing up in a particular family, in a particular region or state, at a particular time. Much of our larger life culture is tacit and relatively inaccessible to easy modification. This is not true of more local cultures, such as in the cockpit of an airliner, or a Navy Seal team, or a clinic. A local culture can, within limits, be established and changed consciously. If getting the right people on the team is the first step, then the second step involves setting the structures, values, incentives, and behavioral conventions that result in high-end team function and integrated care. Here are a few things leaders can do to foster team-based care:

- Start small or at least with projects that have a high likelihood of success. More ambitious projects have a better chance after teams have become a little more accustomed

to the strategies, techniques, and tricks of working together in a complex adaptive system.
- Extensive onboarding. Members naturally work together better when they know each other and know what each other's jobs are. Moreover, shadowing each other through the daily workflow naturally raises potential improvements and solutions even to problems that are not on the problem-solving block right now. Onboarding is insufficient until each team member can describe the job description, competencies, and workday of every other team member.
- Invest in training. The need to put staff "on the floor" for productivity often compromises adequate education and learning over the long term. Lack of knowledge and understanding results in errors, inefficient workflows, and poor quality of care. Shortchanging training almost always results in inefficiencies, errors, and compromised team performance over time.
- Support and promote communication. Team care breaks down fast unless time and other resources are protected for substantive, multimodal communication. Do not assume people know how to communicate with each other. In fact, communication styles and thresholds for information sharing vary dramatically. A psychiatrist may become frustrated when medications are changed by the primary care medical clinician. A primary care clinician is surprised to learn that a patient with diabetes and seizures has been diagnosed by the psychologist with a substance use disorder for years. A security guard is alarmed to discover that the addiction medicine clinic has extended its hours until late evening without informing administrative staff. Gather input from your team and set guidelines about:

  1. What to communicate (e.g., patient needs, schedule changes)
  2. How to communicate (e.g., email, verbally, face to face)
  3. When to communicate (e.g., patient updates during daily huddles, clinic updates during weekly staff meeting)
  4. Who to communicate with (e.g., clinical teams, maintenance, and information technology (IT) staff need to know about schedule changes)

Adjust these guidelines to continuously improve communication.

- Reward interesting solutions: The culture of an evolving, problem-solving, complex clinical environment is reinforced if the problems up for solution are displayed. Moreover, the celebration of solutions, particularly from those in the trenches not traditionally associated with leadership roles, encourages others to take on similar responsibilities. Make it a habit of checking in with staff who perform a variety of functions in the system. Ask the front desk staff what they think can be improved in clinical flow. Engage patients in the problem-solving process. Take an experimental approach to "testing" possible solutions. For example, in a situation in which 20-min psychiatric appointments are desired but the appointment software only allows 15-min appointments, a psychiatric nurse suggests "How about we try to schedule three 15 min appointments each hour and leave the last 15 min open?" "How about we try…" is an oft-heard phrase in the halls of high-functioning organizations.
- Flatten hierarchies: A hierarchical organizational structure tends to assume the leader makes the rules, is always right, and has special access to information denied to the rest of us. All of these factors inhibit smart and fast responses. A culture should be encouraged in which team members can respectfully but emphatically disagree with one another, experiential knowledge is accorded special respect, and solutions are rewarded by their usefulness and not their source.
- Cockpit culture: In the cockpit of a commercial airliner, the pilot is the so-called leader, but the navigator has the authority and responsibility to override this authority under certain circumstances. She must speak forcefully and act decisively when her special knowledge of the airplane's status demands it. All team members defer to the special knowledge of all other team members when appropriate.

- A culture of measurement and measurement-based management: A busy clinic is like an airship buffeted in a storm. In the face of shifting winds and impaired visibility, one can remain fixed on the destination only when your position is accurately measured, and deviation triggers an appropriate response. Measure, respond; measure, respond; measure, respond. It is more important that the response come quickly, and subsequent responses be informed by the effects of those previous, than that the response is "right." Many healthcare professionals earned their place by mastering material, answering questions correctly, solving problems well, and otherwise being right. An admission of error can be understood as bad, even disqualifying. But in the world of complex adaptive systems, the ship is always being knocked off true north, and the adjustment is always imperfect or at least temporary. You must measure the deviation accurately, make an adjustment, measure the effect of the correction, make another adjustment, measure again, and so on, continuously. This applies equally to an overall clinic operation and to an individual patient's personal health plan.

Let us take the measurement-based management part of this discussion a little deeper. This is where we come to the most important and unique kind of leadership found in successful integrated clinic systems: adaptive leadership. This is the leadership that all team members and not just designated leaders display. This is where leadership is most conspicuously not concentrated "at the top" but rather distributed across all members of a team. Adaptive leadership occurs when one or more team members take the lead in improving efficiency or quality in a clinic operation or in dealing with a new problem the clinic is facing. All team members must watch the overall clinic operation all the time. They concentrate on the functions they are uniquely responsible for, but always in the context of overall operation and their ultimate goal.

Cultivate Leadership in All Team Members

We mentioned earlier that all team members function as leaders. This does not happen spontaneously. Some team members, particularly those from the ranks of nonprofessional staff, must be coached, coaxed, and otherwise encouraged into adaptive leadership behavior. This section is the heart of this chapter and is a reminder of our initial point: leadership is a function. You have your vision. You have your team. You have your operating principles and incentives in place. You have your templates and guidelines and process maps and assignments. Now wind everything up, open the doors, and begin. Immediately you start having problems. Nothing ever works in the real world like it does on paper. Early detection of difficulties, swift response, and coordinated action rely on engagement, ownership, and accountability for all team members. If a front-desk receptionist, unaware of integration efforts in the "back of the clinic," fails to notice that the appointment software system automatically cancels every behavioral health appointment associated with a medical appointment, then a cascading flow of misunderstandings, errors, and patient complaints ensues for too long before a "manager in charge" finally identifies and addresses the problem. In an informed and empowered team culture, a receptionist is more likely to understand the value of co-occurring medical and behavioral health appointments, be in continuous touch with the back, recognize the flaw in the scheduling system, and quickly bring this to the attention of other support and clinical team members.

Complex Adaptive Leadership in Action

These principles of adaptive leadership have been derived from direct observation of leaders in successful integrated clinics. This section will describe examples of these observations.

Clarify the Purpose

Let us presume you already have a vision and mission. Now you must create the picture for all team members. What does it look like in your daily life? If we brought a video camera into our clinics 1 year from now, what would the film show? An abstract concept remains elusive until made into a concrete illustration for each team member. Once pictured, you must continually reinforce it—remind staff that any particular problem must be solved in a way that brings you closer to realizing your vision and fulfilling your mission. Recall the initial force toward the existing homeostasis. It is during this transition phase that vigilance and reinforcement are most crucial. For example, imagine the following scenario arising in a routine all-clinic meeting. This is a quarterly meeting run by Laura Marker, the practice's medical director. One of the first items of business is to review together the medical problems that clinic attendees need help with and the adequacy of the practice's response to those problems.

> Laura: "In looking over our clinic's diagnoses for the last three months, we see an alarming new trend. Of the 612 babies we have delivered in this time, 20 have been born addicted to narcotics. I know this doesn't surprise you, since we have already talked a lot about what a terrible problem this is. Not only is it horrible for the infant and mother, but neither we nor our hospital are equipped to deal with this. Our doctors and midwives are way out of their comfort zones, the newborn nursery can't cope with these desperately sick babies, the nearest NICU is three hours away, we don't have a neonatologist on staff, the postpartum floor is overwhelmed, our social workers say the homes they return to are unsafe and unhealthy, and the postpartum calls and visits to our clinic are overwhelming. What are we going to do about this?"
>
> After much discussion about trying to hire a high-risk obstetrician, redoubling efforts to transport out, screening better, more aggressive postpartum follow-up, and a host of other useful but piecemeal solutions, Laura said the following:
>
> "Remember that we are here to help the people in our community be as healthy as they possibly can, no matter what problems they are facing. Therefore, these patients are our problem, and our responsibility. You have already said as much in this meet-

ing, by trying to figure out how we can take better care of people with this overwhelming problem. I think it's time to say that as a practice, we will deal with this problem head-on, and do whatever we have to do to make sure every child born in this county has as good a start in life as possible. This means that we have to reorganize to deal with the opiates in our community, with prevention and treatment; to find and treat all pregnant women who are using as soon as possible; to figure out how to care for neonatal withdrawal syndrome in a small community hospital, to beef up our connection to our referral hospital, and to give these families extra medical and psychosocial attention. This is a tall order. Let's break this up into parts, make assignments among our staff leads, start meeting with our key partners like the hospital CEO, the head of county social services, the police department, and public health. We will also need someone to begin looking at how we can most efficiently accommodate the increased clinical load these patients have brought to the practice. We'll organize the teams to work on this right after this meeting, and you can find others who might want to join later. I'll make sure that all the teams working on this problem have the resources they need to put together a plan of attack by next month. OK, from now until we get a grip on this thing, we will develop some sort of message about 'This is where you come for addiction during pregnancy,' and something for the community about 'Opiates affect everyone's health.' "

Among other things, this is an example of administrative leadership, insofar as Laura called out the problem, lined it up with the clinic's mission, spoke that mission out clearly, and made resources available to go to work on the problem. Note that she left it for those working in the affected areas, those closest to the ground, to more fully characterize the problems and to begin formulating solutions—as adaptive leaders.

Find, Cultivate, and Align Resources

Bring together people, support infrastructure, and funding to implement the vision. It is not just the usual people. Leaders will emerge from *everywhere!*

1. Identify and nurture people who have capacity and discipline to lead, influence, and manage this change process. Identifying leaders can be challenging, as more often than not true leaders do not proclaim their status to you in

boardrooms or executive meetings. We urge you to go to the clinic areas and watch. Observe who people turn to for decision-making, support, and guidance, particularly in ambiguous situations. People choose their leaders. Look for who they are choosing.

2. "Get out of people's way." Enable these identified people, share control, provide structure while protecting flexibility: "Here's my intention; you guys figure out how to do it." There is absolute authority in knowing your job. Ironically, this is one of the most difficult tasks for a leader. Almost every good leader can identify circumstances in which they may have acted differently than the person they assigned to address a problem. It is natural for a leader to want to intervene and "fix problems" for others. Unfortunately, over-functioning for others typically results in under-functioning, demoralization, and relinquished control by key members of your team.

3. Engage everyone at every level. Include people from finance, operations, and clinical teams. Consider again the interdependence and complementarity of all components of a system. Imagine a scenario in which a pediatric medical clinician wishes to add a screening tool for trauma to child wellness visits. This decision affects (a) the office administrative staff who must make multiple copies of the screening form to include in all wellness visit packets, (b) the receptionist who must remember to include the form in all paperwork given to families during wellness visits, (c) the nurse who must collect and enter results into the patient's chart, (d) the psychologist who must review and respond to positive trauma screens, (e) the IT staff who must create electronic fields in the chart for the trauma form results, (f) the coding and billing department who must now include this added screening to the services provided, (g) the finance staff who must consider the added resources (e.g., staff time) in the cost of a wellness visit, and (h) the schedulers who must now accommodate additional time in the appointment for the trauma screening and follow-up. Without education and input at all levels and components of the process, attending to a clinical issue as

important as trauma can be overshadowed and discarded quickly. The implementation of this new quality improvement effort for children is best begun with a meeting of all the aforementioned team members to plan the workflow adjustments it will trigger.

Promote and Reinforce "Transformation Friendly" Behaviors and Practices

1. Celebrate success and embrace failure. While the term "failure" is often viewed as a negative outcome of a decision or event, we think of failure as an incomplete adjustment on the path to improvement and growth. Reframing "failure" as "growth" frees us from the impossible expectations of a positive outcome for every attempt and opens up possibilities for creative, iterative solutions. Take for instance the attempts of an integrated prenatal clinic to develop an appointment template for their high-risk obstetric patients with opiate addictions. An initial attempt at the traditional 8 a.m., 8:15 a.m., 8:30 a.m., etc. schedule results in morning no-shows until about 10 a.m. The prenatal clinic team, frustrated with slow mornings followed by hectic afternoon visits that stretched into the evening, modified the template to schedule four women in 1-hour blocks (four scheduled at 8 a.m., four at 9 a.m., etc.) to allow for flexibility. After 3 months, show rates for prenatal appointments had improved only slightly. Undeterred, the prenatal clinic team carefully reviewed their appointment cycle times, clinician schedules, spoke with the community health coordinators, and, most importantly, asked the pregnant women, "What gets in the way of coming to your visits here?" The pregnant patients cited morning sickness, transportation barriers, conflicts with their addiction treatment, and emotional stress as contributing factors to their poor engagement in prenatal care. It was only after multiple trials with poor outcomes that the prenatal clinic hit on the solution of offering afternoon group prenatal visits co-led

by the psychologist and obstetric physician, including substance abuse treatment and support for transportation. The initial setbacks experienced by the prenatal clinic could be viewed as separate failures or a part of the growth process of a clinic striving to meet the needs of its patients.
2. Live in continuous beta. Beta versions of software are released with the understanding that it still contains bugs that need to be uncovered and fixed. Outline evaluation metrics (process and outcome) and monitor them frequently, using them to refine, stay, or change course. Be nimble — anticipate problems and barriers and be prepared for the unexpected. We turn again to the concept of dynamic equilibrium in a clinic system: change is an expected, necessary, and positive demand on the system. Leaders learn to balance the need for adjustments while staying focused on the mission of the organization. Perhaps more importantly, leaders throughout the team should embrace and exhibit this attitude in the day-to-day work of the clinic. With this perceptual shift, team members absorb the shocks and adjust rather than resist the bumps as disruptions. Practicing in primary care is not a smooth canoe ride over a calm river. It is a thrilling navigation of white water rapids over twists and turns. Act accordingly. In the example above, the continuous efforts to accommodate the needs of addicted pregnant women serve as a good illustration of this principle.
3. Exemplify the model of collaboration, trust, and communication that you are trying to build clinically. People observe and mirror their leaders. If you listen, they are more likely to listen. If you follow through, they are more likely to follow through. A critical role of a leader is to be an anchor for the team, as the team must anchor the patients. The physical, psychological, social, and environmental stressors in the communities we serve are ever-present, chaotic, and constantly threaten the sense of security our patients crave. In bringing behavioral health into the center of primary care practice, we create a space in which people share their most painful struggles. It can feel overwhelming for the

clinic staff to accommodate the changing roles in integration. Being a safe and stable "container" for the reactions and intensity that are inherent in primary care practice is a leadership characteristic with substantial impact throughout the clinic and community at large.
4. Let jobs bleed into each other, and do the job whenever it presents. One of the most corrosive things you can hear in a busy clinic is "That's not my job." In contrast, supporting a culture in which people share functions in service of a collective goal reinforces the focus on the mission and interdependence between team members. The multifaceted nature of primary care all but guarantees that numerous tasks, unexpected and unassigned, will emerge and must be completed. A patient speaking an unknown language shows up in the clinic. A community health worker walking by stops and tries to communicate with the patient with written symbols and hand gestures. A pipe leak leaves a puddle of water on the bathroom floor. The pharmacist finds a mop and cleans the floor. The receptionist becomes ill and a therapist helps answer phones. Reward people who step up and respond to problems without being asked. Model doing what needs to be done.

Lead the Actual Transformation Effort

When a primary care clinic begins the transformation into an integrated clinic, with a behavioral health clinician working as part of the core primary care team, clinic operations and patient workflows will necessarily change. Let us imagine that a full-time clinical psychologist is added to the clinic schedule in a four-primary care provider (PCP) practice. Let us further imagine that this person has already negotiated the details of her position description and intends to divide her time into three equal parts: she will be available to offer psychotherapy for mental disorders, will directly help patients with their chronic disease self-management programs, and will also be available for real-time consultations and warm handoffs. She will also facilitate referral to specialty care for psychiatric emergencies and severe psychiatric conditions. Concurrent with this hire, the clinic begins screening every patient in the waiting room with the PHQ-9, expecting that the psychologist will see all the patients who meet criteria for major depression. Clinic leaders may draft the workflow changes their clinic will need to make, but it is just not possible even for experienced clinics to anticipate everything that will need to change to accommodate a new resource such as this. It is up to the team on the ground, the ones doing the actual clinical work, to lead with ideas, proposals, and rapid-cycle changes to restore equilibrium and clinical function at a higher level. Several examples will illustrate how this works.

1. Positive PHQs accrue at the rate of 16 per week. The psychologist initiates an eight-session CBT program for four new patients per week and coaches the PCPs to manage the others themselves. At the end of 2 months, when she reaches equilibrium, she is doing 32 hours of CBT a week and is unavailable for most of the other parts of her job description. At the next clinical team meeting, attended by the appointment clerk, the care manager, four medical assistants (MAs), a clinical pharmacist, and the four PCPs, the PCPs all agree that this is not the best use of the psychologist, and they want to free her up to accept warm handoffs and see patients in distress who might not meet criteria for depression. They agree that only the most severely depressed patients, and only those who express a clear preference for psychotherapy, will be scheduled to see the psychologist. She agrees to reduce the one-on-one work to 12 hours a week. The team explores the possibility of group psychotherapy sessions, but temporarily rejects this idea for scheduling and other logistical reasons.
2. At the second team meeting after the psychologist is on board, the MA presents her depression phone follow-up log, which shows that she has contacted only half the patients the protocol calls for. She cannot add all these calls to her other responsibilities. The appointment clerk

says her call burden is relatively light from 10 am to noon most days, and she could make some of these calls if she were trained in motivational interviewing and had a list of appropriate questions to ask. The team agrees that this is a good use of the scheduling clerk, and this training occurs.
3. The depression screening results in a significant number of new patients on antidepressants that are managed by the PCPs, and much of this is uncomfortable for them—they feel like they are practicing beyond their competence. The clinical pharmacist offers to do an inservice on the use of antidepressants and to monitor the charts of all patients on these drugs for effectiveness and safety. This is a most welcome suggestion that is implemented immediately.
4. The scheduling clerk describes a scheduling problem for the psychologist. Patients want more availability in the afternoons, particularly mid-week. The PCPs, on the other hand, are complaining that they need the psychologist to be available for curbside consults and warm handoffs on Mondays and Fridays when they see more walk-ins and acute patients. The scheduling clerk proposes to schedule the psychologist more heavily on Tuesday, Wednesday, and Thursday afternoons and leave her relatively unscheduled (and therefore available to the PCPs) on Mondays and Fridays. This turns out to be a splendid solution.

There is a continuous stream of problems like this with scheduling, communication, shared clinical plans, and other details of workflow and clinical care that a properly authorized and resourced team can manage themselves. These clinical team members are adaptive leaders, and the operation of an advanced integrated clinic absolutely depends on their leadership. The administrative leaders need to stay out of their way but also need to know what they are attempting, what succeeds and what does not, and need to track whether solutions are producing the kind of care that lines up with their mission. These administrative (and facilitative leaders) also need to make sufficient resources available for the adaptive leaders to work with.

Things to Put on the Wall

This section is to point out that we all need reminders and to give specific examples of what we need to be reminded of. What do we aspire to become? Why we are here? What we are here to do? How we operate? What do we value? What are our rules of the road? This is singing the same song together in order to become a choir. There are many ways to do this. Many clinics hang sayings on the walls of hallways, break rooms, and exam rooms. Epigraphs on email templates can work. Pushing out to all staff a Saying-a-Day can work. Opening every meeting with a recitation of mission, or vision, or values, or taglines, or other relevant statements is a powerful reminder of purpose. This aligns the work on specific problems with overall goals.

You remind yourself of not just those eternal truths but also reflect on where your organization is at the moment. For example, think about the conflict continuum. At one end, conflict is so low that everyone agrees with the leader or with each other. There is no critical thinking, and the best ideas and solutions never get surfaced. At the other extreme conflict is so savage and toxic, so ad hominem, that it harms people and inhibits participation and trying new ideas. You want your team to have spirited disagreements with one another on the way to finding the best ideas, but not so sharp that they hurt or inhibit each other. If your team is too agreeable, too groupthink, you may need a saying on the wall like "For every idea, surface a different idea. Diversity of opinion rules!" For a group that attacks and backbites and undermines each other's ideas, you might want to post something like: "Respect each other. Encourage the voice of those who speak least." If your team is too agreeable and nonconfrontational, a saying like "Challenge everything" might be more helpful.

Your wall sayings need to change from time to time. Someone, or maybe a communications team, should be responsible for this. There are some things that pretty much inspire and instruct no matter what, but many sayings are more or less helpful according to where you are along the conflict continuum, or risk-avoidance continuum, or planning-flexibility continuum, or over- under-communication continuum, or long-range-short-range continuum. Here are a few examples we have taken from walls, table tents, epigraphs, and other places around successful integrated clinics.

- Remember why we are here: to help people become a little healthier.
- Expect problems. Welcome them as a sign that we are alive.
- Speak up. Speak the truth and have no fear.
- Be kind. Kindness trumps cleverness every time.
- Try something, anything, then fine-tune it. Life is a beta test.
- Listen closely to what people say and how they say it. Write the best of it down.
- Be cold and objective in judging whether it works. In the world of actual things, nothing works perfectly, and nothing works forever.
- Do not let little problems persist. Small nagging problems corrode morale. Fix them.
- The hard stuff we do right away. It is the impossible stuff that takes a little time.
- Bite off more than you can chew. Then offer—*offer*—some of it to your neighbor.
- Conflict is good. Not war, conflict. It brings people together.
- Let yourself be disturbed but not abused.
- A lot of the time, you are just wrong. It is a sign of taking a position. Own it.
- Set things right before they arise. Anticipate problems. Have a long time horizon.
- Unless we go to extremes, we will never get anywhere. Tackle hard problems, and try radical solutions. Solve hard.
- Expect surprises. This is not an oxymoron.
- Sometimes the answers lie outside our world.
- Get in the mix. Let your partners disturb your ideas. Too much time behind a closed door is bad.

- That fix is temporary. No matter how well it works, it will only work for so long.
- You are the best person to do certain jobs. Do those jobs. Do what nobody but you can do.
- Be stable but flexible. This is not an oxymoron.
- Yes, you are a kid in a candy store. Learn things. Try stuff. Enjoy yourself. But remember: candy is not one of the basic food groups. We have work to do around here.
- Plan but be spontaneous. This is not an oxymoron.
- Respect your partners and celebrate their successes.
- Did it make our patients healthier?
- Never stop thinking about how to do it better.

The Elevator Speech

It helps for those who are building transformed, integrated practices to be able to say, clearly and succinctly, *what* they are doing, *why* they are doing it, and *how* to do it. These "elevator speeches" can be delivered in 15–30 seconds, the time it takes to pass between floors on an elevator. They are for external and internal consumption alike. On the one hand, they inspire supporters and partners; on the other hand, they galvanize and concentrate an organization's sense of purpose and direction. The principles and practices of leadership described in this chapter are useful as templates or starters for leaders who wish to craft elevator speeches. Of course a brief description of what you are doing, or why, or how will vary according to your audience. With that caveat in mind, here is a sample of elevator speeches designed to answer the following questions:

1. "What are you working on these days?"

"We're still in the business of trying to improve the health of the people in our three-county area, and we're still trying to do that by offering high-quality primary care. Right now we are integrating behavioral healthcare into our primary care clinics, so we can address most or all of our patients' healthcare needs onsite. This is comprehensive, integrated care, and we think it will help our patients be healthier." It takes about 20 seconds to say this paragraph. You may wish to adjust this to better fit the particulars of your mission or to emphasize other elements, such as the coordination effort, or prevention, or community engagement, or longitudinal care – whatever your particular efforts are at the time.

2. "Why are you doing that?"

"Well, we know there are a few things that reliably improve the quality of primary care, and two of them are comprehensiveness and coordination of care. We can win big improvements in both of those by incorporating attention to behavioral concerns into every visit. Besides, the patients love it. So do the PCPs – they won't go back to the old way." Again, adjust according to your audience and the particular features that you are actually addressing.

3. "How do you do this?"

"The first thing we have done is to hire behavioral health clinicians for every clinic – enough so that every patient has access to one. The next thing is that we are learning to practice in teams, instead of in a one-on-one fashion. We are also measuring a lot more stuff – the quality of our care, our health outcomes – and making many more adjustments to improve our processes and outcomes. We've had to rethink all of our practice habits and beliefs to continuously improve. After an initial rough start, now everybody prefers this new way of practicing."

Practice transformation is difficult but rewarding. It is impossible without active leadership. This chapter has highlighted a few of the most salient features of leadership that one sees in successfully integrated clinical systems.

Additional Reading

Cannon W. The wisdom of the body: how the body reacts to disturbance and danger and maintains the stability essential to life. New York: Norton; 1932.

Heifitz R, Grashow A, Linsky M. The practice of adaptive leadership: tools and tactics for changing your organization and the world. Cambridge, MA: Harvard Business Review Press; 2009.

Lencioni P. Overcoming the five dysfunctions of a team: a field guide. San Francisco: Jossey-Bass; 2005.

McChrystal S, Collins T, Silverman D, Fussell C. Team of teams: new rules of engagement for a complex world. New York: Portfolio/Penguin; 2015.

Schmitz P. Everyone leads: building leadership from the community up. San Francisco: Jossey Bass; 2012.

Tzu L. Tao Te Ching. ~500 BC. Translated by S. Mitchell. New York: Harper Collins; 1988.

Chapter 6
It Takes a Team

F. Alexander Blount

Preamble

Team-based values, methods, and relationships are now ubiquitous in conversation about primary care. Everyone values "team" and claims to be doing it in one form or another—or having done it all along—"nothing new for me." But what is the substance underlying the slogan? What are the benefits to adding a behavioral health (BH) clinician as a long-missing member of the primary care team? How can you deploy behavioral health clinicians to achieve these benefits? What are the properties of different models of integration? How can you be clear enough about this new role to effectively interview and hire for it? In other words, how can this role be truly integrated functionally, not just "anatomically"? *CJP*

F. A. Blount
Department of Clinical Psychology, Antioch University New England, Keene, NH, USA

Department of Family Medicine and Psychiatry, University of Massachusetts Medical School, Amherst, MA, USA

Introduction

"Team care" is all the rage these days. Primary care doctors are all being urged to adopt it, if they have not already.[1] But who can blame a doctor for thinking, "I've had a team all along. You think I make all the appointments, check people in, put patients in rooms, take their vitals, prepare procedure trays, give shots, change exam rooms, and check people out all by myself?" The question that this doctor has to face is, "With all that help, why is it that you still feel so stressed?" The doctor has been imagining that with one more medical assistant, or with two fewer patients a day, it would be comfortable again.

Many of his or her colleagues who have been working in high functioning teams would disagree. They would say that their stress has been reduced because other members of the team are handling elements of a visit that the doctor alone used to handle. Perhaps even more, those doctors would say that now they are giving more complete and effective treatment to patients with behavioral health (BH) issues that previously were not adequately addressed. Those patients used to come back more often because their care was not addressing their needs. That meant that the patients that the doctors felt least effective in treating gradually took up more and more of their daily schedule.

The same doctors who are practicing in high-functioning teams would also tell you that the transition was not easy or quick. Not every member of the group of staff working with each doctor, and for that matter, not every doctor, wants to evolve their roles in delivering care to patients. The changes involve more time meeting together and looking at issues like mission and values in addition to workflows and assignments. We will talk about this process in more detail later.

Adding a "behavioral health clinician," a psychologist or clinical social worker or another licensed counselor who is additionally trained to work in primary care, adds more than one more body to the team. The new staff member, whom I will call a BH clinician, adds a new expertise set, a new way of

---

[1] I prefer to call PCPs "doctors" because that is usually what their patients call them, whether they are MD, DO, NP, or PA.

approaching problems, and a way of addressing issues patients face that previously were sources of frustration and failure for the patients and their doctors. One of the first outcomes that has been identified when BH clinicians first join medical practices as team members is that "provider satisfaction" goes up [3]. Doctors tend to feel relieved and supported in new ways. They are not carrying the whole load of knowing what to do in all their most complex cases, and they are not feeling that they are inadequately serving the many anxious and depressed patients that present every day, usually presenting with complaints the patients experience as medical.

Deploying a BH Clinician

So, for a little while, let us imagine that you solve the issues of funding and you are able to hire a BH clinician for your practice. What do you do with him or her to get this "provider satisfaction" and better patient care? In deciding how to deploy a BH clinician, think about the problem you most want to solve. Would you like to focus on getting treatment to more of your patients? Is there a population of patients in your practice, e.g., people with depression or poorly managed diabetes, that you would like to be the target of your new resource? Finally, in addition to having more of your patients seen, would you like to have your new colleague available for convenient consultation in the flow of care? How you answer these questions will make the difference in whether you decide to pursue a "co-located" arrangement, a Collaborative Care approach, or Primary Care Behavioral Health (PCBH) model initially. If you are like most places, you will gradually evolve a hybrid that works best in your setting.

Co-location Model

A first step in many sites is an arrangement called "co-location." This arrangement locates a BH clinician *doing therapy, in the primary care office suite, by referral* from the doctor or group of doctors who practice in those offices. It requires a little quiet space somewhere in the suite, but nothing more fancy. It will be important to have the BH clinician documenting in the EMR so that the behavioral health diagnoses, observations, and progress made by the patient and BH clinician can be in the front of the doctor's mind when he or she sees the patient next.

This co-location arrangement goes a long way toward solving one problem and may solve a second. It greatly improves the options for referrals to some sort of mental health or substance use disorder treatment, because patients will accept care by a professional in a primary care office much more readily than they will go to a separate mental health facility or private practitioner. Your success rate of referrals (meaning the patient has at least one visit with the new resource) will likely change in the general range from 20–30% for outside referrals to 70–80% or more for inside referrals if your practice is typical of the many I have talked to. Just knowing so many people are now getting seen is a load off your mind.

Coordinating with your BH clinician in providing care, an arrangement in which you prescribe psychotropic medication for depression or anxiety or attention-deficit disorder and the BH clinician maintains closer contact, teaching coping skills, and offering therapy can be a much more satisfying approach to practice than trying to refer patients to outside resources. Most doctors feel they can be more judicious in the use of medications once they have a BH clinician as part of the team for patients. This puts them more comfortably within the evidence-based recommendations. In the case of depression, for instance, some degree of depression is extremely common and impacts the health and functioning of a great many people. It is only in the case of depression that meets criteria for major depressive disorder that medication is one of the evidence-based choices and only in the case of severe depression that medication is strongly recommended [7].

A challenge that you can face in a co-located arrangement is that it tends to make the BH clinician define psychotherapy as their main job. If they have not had sufficient training to know how to move beyond the kinds of therapies they were doing in a mental health facility (we will talk a lot more about training later), they may initiate that kind of therapy in most cases. That means they would engage patients in longer-term approaches to therapy, meaning more visits, and each visit would take up an hour, between talking and writing the note. This leads to the BH clinician's schedule filling up. After your initial relief at being able to find care for so many of your patients for whom a referral did not work previously, you can end up with an internal waiting list. It is very frustrating to want care for a patient and have the BH clinician in your office tell you that the patient can be seen in 3 or 4 weeks. For co-location to work in a busy practice, the length of each visit will need to be shorter, probably not longer than a half hour, and the mean number of visits in an episode of care will be around three. This is possible if the BH clinician can make an adaptation from the reflective types of therapies many are taught for mental health specialty work to a more targeted, problem-focused approach [8]. Treatment focused on a problem creates a different expectation for patients as opposed to treatment that is thought of as "beginning therapy." In that case, treatment only goes as long as patients think they need to come. Patients tend to come until they notice improvement and then they have better things to do with the time and the money [2]. In this model, that is allowed, as is returning when they feel they need a bit more help.

Collaborative Care Model

If you choose to bring on a BH clinician to address the needs of a specific population in your office, you will probably be implementing a Collaborative Care approach. This is an approach with strong evidence for clinical outcomes for patients [11]. It was developed as a variation of the Chronic Care Model [12], a variation that targeted depression as the chronic disease. The Collaborative Care approach is built on reliable identification of the group of your patients who make up the population, usually by using a screening tool such as the PHQ-9. Reliable identification, in this approach, leads to the offering to all (or as many as possible) of the members of the population an evidence-based protocol of treatment. Finally, it includes active monitoring of adherence, side effects, and effectiveness throughout the course of treatment, with additional intensity of care offered to patients for whom the initial treatment protocol does not seem to be effective. Since a brief targeted dose of therapy (four to eight visits in various implementations of the model) is one of the choices in an evidence-based protocol for most patients, your BH clinician will be your provider for this element. A slight majority of patients who have less than severe depression tend to prefer the "counseling" intervention over medication as a first step [4]. The monitoring of adherence, side effects, and effectiveness can be done by the BH clinician in addition to providing therapy, though some practices use lesser trained staff, who still need specific training for this role, to ask the questions when patients come for visits and to make telephone calls between visits.

Options for additional intensity of care, or "stepped care," need to be part of the Collaborative Care Model for the patients who do not respond adequately to the initial protocol [6]. Sometimes this involves a pre-arranged referral arrangement with a nearby mental health facility. More commonly, it involves the possibility of more visits with the BH clinician, on one hand, and a more complex approach to medication, on the other. For this, having access to consultation with a psychiatrist or expert psychiatric nurse practitioner is important. In many cases, doctors do not feel comfortable taking on an approach such as Collaborative Care without regular consultation and discussion with the psychiatrist. Most, but not all of the studies of the Collaborative Care Model, have used psychiatrists to support or guide the process from the beginning. Some used psychologists for the clinical consultation and psychiatrists to consult on prescribing [11]. Over time, the doctors tend to gain more confidence in their own prescribing expertise and can use the psychiatrist to help with more unusual stepped care cases.

The advantages of the Collaborative Care approach are many. As in other approaches, a lot of patients who otherwise would not get care are given treatment. It is a clearly outlined approach, so the uncertainty about how to implement the new program is reduced. Roles of various team members are clearly prescribed. It fits with the data gathered by quality measures commonly used by the government, other payers and with accreditation measures of the National Committee for Quality Assurance (NCQA) and other certifying agencies.

The disadvantages of the Collaborative Care approach are that, without some modification, it tends to keep the doctor and BH clinician on different tracks during the flow of care. The BH clinician is providing prescribed "doses" of therapy or doing monitoring of current patients and is not easily available to doctors for consultation. It can also be frustrating to doctors and to patients that a behavioral health service is operating in the practice, but the population being addressed is by no means the entire group of patients who need behavioral health intervention. The author visited one community health center in which the provider group had abandoned their formal Collaborative Care program for exactly this reason. The doctors could not justify involving a resource for patients with one diagnosis and not being able to offer the resource to patients they judged to be just as disabled by other behavioral health disorders. They developed their own approach that allowed much more "doctor discretion" about which patients were seen by the BH clinicians, while maintaining the screening program, the protocols of brief care, and the monitoring implemented when the Collaborative Care approach was launched. Finally, the Collaborative Care Model has shown much better results in controlled studies than in broader implementations. In a state-wide implementation in Minnesota called the DIAMOND Project supported by specially designed payment models, participating clinics delivered more elements of the model and showed better patient satisfaction than usual care, but depression remission rates were no higher than nonparticipating clinics [10].

Primary Care Behavioral Health Model

The last way of deploying your BH clinician as a resource is called the Primary Care Behavioral Health (PCBH) model. It is also sometimes called the Behavioral Health Consultant (BHC) model. The word "Consultant" is used in the title to remind doctors and BH clinicians that, where possible, the goal of the approach is to maintain the patient's experience that their doctor is in the lead of their care and to help the doctor in the many ways that someone with strong behavioral health expertise can to enhance the care they provide. This can be done through targeted brief interventions and by offering consultation on diagnoses, needs, and possibilities for patients in the flow of the doctor's care.

In this approach, the BH clinician becomes part of the infrastructure of the practice, used for a quick opinion or added to the care of some patients at the doctor's discretion (augmented by screening). Instead of referring patients to the BH clinician for care, or adding them to a pre-set program for a population, the BH clinician is involved in their care for whatever seems needed at the time. As an example, you could ask the BH clinician to speak to the patient in exam room A to see if he or she thinks the patient's obvious dysphoria is part of a picture that warrants further treatment at this time and if the treatment would be best offered by the doctor, the BH clinician, both, or some other service. You could ask for an opinion in another case about why an obviously intelligent patient has steadfastly failed to adhere to a medical regimen that could prolong his or her life, despite the doctor's best efforts to make the situation clear to him or her. You could ask the BH clinician to teach another patient a technique that allows people to put themselves to sleep more easily, as a first-level intervention for insomnia. If you think about all the times in the day when you wish for a quick consult or intervention on psychosocial or behavioral issues, you can think of a lot of ways that a BH clinician in this model could make your life easier. This does not have to add a lot of time to your day. The BH clinician can meet with one patient while you go on to another.

The use of your BH clinician as an internal consultant has all the advantages of improved access plus patient and provider satisfaction of the co-located approach. In fact, this is the approach that gets some behavioral health expertise and care added to the overall care of the largest portion of your patients. It would logically follow that if this approach engages a BH clinician with the most patients, no matter how efficiently the engagement is effected, it is also the approach that would require the most BH clinicians for a busy practice. The ratio of BH clinicians is variable depending on the acuity of the population, how sophisticated the doctors are at using them in the flow care, and how comfortable the BH clinician is at addressing chronic illnesses and health behavior change needs. If all of these are high (acuity, sophistication, and generalism), probably one full-time BH clinician could adequately support two to three full-time doctors as a start.

The benefits to the doctors and for other medical team members are more support and more teaming in the flow of care. Over time the medical team members gain more behavioral health expertise and tend to practice more "behaviorally enhanced" medicine though they do not begin doing the work of the BH clinician. This approach is also very exciting and interesting to the BH clinicians that choose it. And "choose it" is important here. In programs in which clinicians from a mental health organization have been assigned to work in a primary care setting, they often are very unhappy. A BH clinician has to enjoy the fast pace and the uncertainty of what each patient encounter will bring in primary care. Those for whom that style is a fit, usually in the behavioral health consultant role, become happy and confident team members. They often get assigned other new roles in the organization that need confidence, creativity, and flexibility.

The other side of the flexibility coin is that these clinicians have had to make the most adaptation to primary care culture and practice patterns from their original training in specialty mental health therapies. Mental health graduate training is usually built on the idea that medical and behavioral health constitute different worlds of diagnosis and care. The need to make the adaptation to providing primary care behavioral health tends to select for personal flexibility and being able to function confidently within the uncertainties of primary care practice.

The challenges of the PCBH model tend to be those attendant to an approach that is less bound to the prevailing assumptions and practice patterns that are the basis for the "diagnose, treat, bill" sequence in the fee-for-service payment world. On the other hand, the more a practice goes to bundled payments or shared risk payment model, the more the flexibility of this approach, and the people who are schooled in it, will stand in good stead when it comes to sustainability.

Hiring

Your first BH clinician may be the most important hire of your new team. It is probably easiest to say who you do not want. The leaders from the ACT implementation in Colorado (a large multi-site implementation of behavioral health integration; see description in Chap. 1), the researchers who studied behavioral health integration in exemplar practices for the Agency for Healthcare Research and Quality (AHRQ) Integration Academy, and most of the other leaders in the movement to develop the primary care behavioral health workforce agree that you do not want a BH clinician (psychiatrist, psychologist, social worker, or counselor) who has only been trained in and only worked in specialty mental health [5]. This is a challenge, because very few of the graduate training programs in the US are training clinicians to work in primary care. Most who learn these skills in their degree programs learn them in experiential training placements in primary care. There are some very good programs available online as post-degree transition training, such as the primary care behavioral health training program of the Center for Integrated Primary Care at the University of Massachusetts Medical School, and the guild organizations, such as the American Psychological Association and the American Psychiatric Association, have developed programs and curricula. There are a growing number of primary care health settings that offer practicums, internships, or post-doctoral fellowships for BH clinicians in training that help students make the transition to primary care culture and methods. The change offered by an organized training program is as much cultural as it is skill based, so a workshop or two in skills alone tends not to be sufficient. You do not want an "untrained" person if there is an alternative.

If you do not have the option of hiring someone who has worked in primary care or has trained for primary care, hire on the basis of personality. You are looking for someone who is open to learning, who sees working in primary care as a unique opportunity rather than as a less than rigorous mental health delivery setting. You want someone who is comfortable with generalism, who is interested in seeing the full range of patients in your practice, someone who makes friends with other staff members easily, and who likes the idea of other staff members helping out with the behavioral treatment load in some way rather than a professional who spends energy patrolling disciplinary boundaries and arguing about who is qualified to do what. You want somebody who is expected to do what is necessary for a patient, such as some elements of care management, rather than someone who takes an "it's not my job" approach. When you are interviewing candidates, do not ask them if they work in the way just described. Ask them to tell you a clinical story in which they look good and look to see which of these qualities you can see in the story. You can ask the same question for an organizational story. Have them tell a story where there was some difficulty or issue in an organization where they worked and how they kept it from getting worse or contributed to making it better. Push for enough detail so you can visualize the interaction, and if you find it impossible to visualize the patient and their situation that are being described in your candidate's story because of psychological vagueness or jargon, e.g., "I did CBT," you can be confident that you will have a hard time working on a collaborative clinical team with this person. If the patient(s) come across as understandable human beings in the story, and the interventions described make sense to you, e.g., "I worked with her to pick one thing she could do every day that she enjoyed and we tracked those for the next two weeks," that is a very good indication. The more your candidate includes an understanding of the patient's family and other elements of their context, such as their culture, in designing treatment approaches, the more their expertise likely will be understandable and helpful to other team members.

Hiring other members of the team when you need to is probably more familiar. For most of these roles, medical or administrative skills need to be in place. For these roles, the behavioral skills needed in the job are called "people skills."

Look for people who find ways to relate positively to patients, who are interested in patients' stories. See if you can find people who have some hope of sharpening their own skills, who want to earn the right to take on increased responsibility appropriate to their training. In the long run, you will want everyone to be able to do some motivational interviewing to help patients improve their health by changing their health behaviors.

Building Team Culture

Over time a successful team creates a culture that is durable, not dependent only on the attitudes and practice style of the doctor. The addition of the BH clinician to the team begins this process by adding an expertise set to the team that is separate from and additional to the expertise of the doctor. For the first time, the doctor is asking a team member for clinical input, not just for assistance. It is a profound and usually unheralded moment. This begins opening space for the whole team to see how the team can be "smarter" than any one member without losing its coherence or leadership. As the doctor, you might find that some team members have the same degree of challenges to working in this new team as you. They can be reticent about sharing what they know or what they think because of their experience of doctors who were not interested in their observations and opinions. If they are like many of their peers, they will wait for the doctor to set the agenda, to tell them what to do. Over time, as team members get more comfortable accessing multiple expertise sets, there is one more set of expertise that is available and that can be transformative: the expertise of the patient.

You might want to consider having a "mission talk" that you deliver at your first team meeting after your BH clinician is hired. It is a brief statement that expresses the mission of the team. It should be fairly brief, a conversation you bring up in essentially the same form whenever a new member of the team is added.

The message can describe the patient as the center of the team's efforts and as a full team member in their own care, whose knowledge and preferences are fundamental to designing their treatment plan. It is sensible every time to highlight the way that behavioral health is "mission critical" to the team. You might want to say something about how team members value each other's special relationships with and therefore special knowledge of patients. It could be worth saying that we watch each other for signs of stress or struggle and show caring when we see them. The talk should encourage each team member being able to articulate the roles of all team members to patients and to other people. And it should support learning from each other and being able to cover for each other in situations in which the coverage is clearly appropriate and boundaries of licensure are respected. After a few deliveries, you hope that the talk will be so familiar to the team that when a new team member starts on a day when you cannot be at the meeting, other members deliver the talk because they have heard it so many times. This is how you build a culture over time that is self-sustaining.

Communication in the Team

Ongoing communication within the team is vital for team functioning, both at regular meetings for predictable communication and through brief exchanges of information to keep each other up to date in the flow of care. For regular meetings, some practices have one meeting a week to address a range of matters, and other practices have more than one kind of meeting and address different sorts of issues at different times. Some have longer meetings to get it all done, while some have briefer meetings because those are more efficient for them. It is very hard to say what schedule and organization will work for a practice.

It is a fair generalization that primary care practices, and medical services in general, have so much to do that they try to have as little time in meetings as possible. This leads to a common situation in which a practice avoids meetings and then has barely enough communication to keep things moving. In this situation, team members are more likely to feel overwhelmed. The idea that more communication is needed to plan changes in workflows, to evaluate the results, do brief targeted training, or to talk about mission or values, and that the investment in more communication could leave everyone less stressed and help the practice provide better care more efficiently, can be a very hard sell. It is also true that time spent in meetings which is not productive or conversations that do not relate to the jobs the team has to accomplish will lead to meetings losing the engagement of team members.

Examples of topics for regularly occurring meetings:

1. One or two patients that team members feel the team could engage or manage better: nonadherent patients, scary patients, dissatisfied patients, patients who are not getting better, and patients with complex lives that need to be understood better.
2. How can we improve? The team looks at data, something that is being counted, and sees where the numbers look good and where there might be a place to try something different. Or they remember together one or two specific instances when things did not go smoothly and think about how those specific situations could be handled better in the future. Before spending too much time looking for a fix, spend some time looking for instances when that same process or task went well. See what various team members did in those instances. Whatever the sequence, it is something they already know how to do and could be the basis for making that success more frequent.
3. Highlight excellence: Take a moment to let team members recite things that other members did that were noticeably helpful, or insightful, or caring, or courageous. Make sure they describe specifically what their teammate did that they appreciated.

It might be good to have a weekly meeting time with rotating topics so that the time is always interesting and useful.

Perhaps the most useful regular meeting is the huddle before each session of patient care. A huddle is a 5–15-min meeting in which all of the people who will be providing or assisting in patient care during the session exchange information that will help everyone work in a coordinated and efficient way. When you first start to hold huddles there will likely be push back. "We could use this time better to each get ready for our individual role." Do not give in. Once they see how much better the half day goes, how much less stressed everyone is, and how much less follow-up work there is, they will come around.

If you are using the BH clinician as a consultant in the flow of care, a huddle is the best way to involve her in the care efficiently and effectively. Look at the schedule. Which patients could use a brief check-in on how they are doing with their depression or anxiety or drinking? The BH clinician can be called in before or after your contact with the patient. Is there a smoker or two that the BH clinician might look in on before you get to them? It is often possible to help a patient move one stage of change toward better health in that time. Then when you come in, the BH clinician and the patient can sum up what they have discussed and what the patient is going to do in 1–2 min, and the BH clinician can leave. You can start your visit with the patient offering support or congratulations. Think about how much more enjoyable those visits would be. For a good deal of more material on building a highly functioning team, see the American Medical Association's "Steps Forward" site at https://www.stepsforward.org/modules/team-based-care.

For help in building a team that includes a BH clinician, see https://www.integration.samhsa.gov/workforce/team-members.

Workflows

Adding your BH clinician and the services he or she contributes to the team will inevitably impact workflows. If you are going to address behavioral health issues in any organized way, you will be doing behavioral health screening of some sort. Workflows in a primary care team are modified by the introduction of screening for BH concerns, such as depression (recommended by the United States Preventive Services Task Force for adults and adolescents), alcohol (recommended for adults), other substance use disorders, anxiety, post-traumatic stress disorder (PTSD), or other concerns that might be relevant to your patient population. You and the BH clinician can decide what screens to use and where to start.

Some practices want to use the most brief sorts of screens comparatively often. With these screens, a positive response has to be followed up by administration of a longer screen to help with diagnosis, which is a workflow challenge. A negative screen, however, takes very little time and needs no further discussion. A longer screen, perhaps given annually, with more frequent administrations to higher risk groups, can be followed up for diagnosis and possible intervention directly without a second step, but it takes more time up front.

You might want to use the decision about how to handle behavioral health screens in the workflow as one to which the whole team can contribute. On most teams, multiple members of the team get involved in distributing, scoring, assessing results, interacting with patients about the results, and confirming diagnoses. The weekly meeting can be a time to launch and evaluate lots of small workflow adjustments. Having the team in on developing workflows should help with follow-through. When everyone is aware of why the new sequence is being tried, that it is being piloted, how it should help or improve some past inefficiency, and that they will have a part in evaluating the results, they are more likely to help with carrying it out.

Take some time discussing the words or phrases that team members will use to describe what a screen is for and how it will be used. Small differences in wording can make a difference in how well patients respond and how open they are to some sort of intervention later. You want to normalize the questions and make the information gained seem to open up the possibility of the team offering more effective care. In my practice, the screening sheet, a collection of standard depression, anxiety, PTSD and alcohol screens, was called "The Patient Stress Questionnaire." People found it to be a reasonable and helpful set of questions. One approach to helping team members do their part in the screening process is to offer scripts for how to introduce a BH screen or respond to a positive screen. When they know what to say, they experience success and the whole area of BH care becomes likely to feel more familiar and related to their work.

The fact that the team has multiple experts in the patients' care means that there probably needs to be more communication about a patient while they are at the practice. Having the conversation about the patient and their care in the exam room with the patient saves time, increases patient engagement and participation, and helps grow the expertise of all the team members.

The practice of having conversations about the patient in the presence of the patient is helpful in integrated primary care settings. It tends to start at the "passing of the relationship" when the doctor wants to add the BH clinician to the care. Without being able to speak in front of the patient this exchange is usually inefficient. It involves a double exchange of information, as when the doctor and BH clinician exchange information about the patient in the hall and then a social introduction between the patient and BH clinician is made in the exam room. It makes starting the new relationship between the BH clinician and the patient somewhat awkward, because the patient does not know what the BH clinician has been told about him or her and the BH clinician has to spend time beginning a conversation and establishing a mutual purpose for the meeting.

When the introduction and exchange of information about the patient are done in the presence of the patient, the existing doctor-patient dyad can be transitioned much more comfortably and effectively into a BH clinician-patient dyad. The "warm handoff" is done in the room with the patient, the BH clinician, and the doctor. The doctor leads. It is an introduction that is designed to make working with the BH clinician maximally acceptable to the patient and to orient the BH clinician to the person and the task.

Consider using the mnemonic of SSRI to organize the passing of the relationship between the doctor and the patient to the patient and the new BH clinician. It is designed to help doctors know how to conduct this process smoothly and efficiently.

The first S is for **Situation.** The doctor says to the patient and the BH clinician what *situation* in the patient's current care makes him or her want to add the BH clinician to the treatment team.

The second S is **Skill Set.** The doctor describes to the patient the *skill set* (as opposed to the discipline) of the BH clinician that makes him or her the person that she wants to add to the treatment team.

The R stands for **Relationship**. At this point, the doctor says what *relationship* the work between the BH clinician and the patient will have to the overall treatment that she has been directing. Remember, this is not a new treatment; it is a new aspect of the patient's current care.

The final I is for **Indicators**. The doctor says to the BH clinician and the patient what would *indicate* that the addition of the BH clinician's expertise and intervention had been successful.

Below are three examples of introductions designed to add a BH clinician to the care of a patient in a way that allows the patient and BH clinician to achieve targeted improvement through an efficient and effective interaction. Notice that the doctor does not specify what sort of intervention the BH clinician will use nor how many contacts between the BH clinician and the patient will be involved. Those are dependent on the expertise of the BH clinician and the connection that develops between clinician and patient.

In each case, there is a social introductory sentence before the SSRI statements. In the first case it would be, "Ms. Ruiz, this is Dr. Collins. Dr. Collins, this is Ms. Ruiz."

> **Situation:** "Ms Ruiz has terrible headaches. I think they may be related to stress."

Skill Set: "Dr. Collins (BH clinician) is an expert at helping people cope with stress."

Relationship: "I am hoping that you and Dr. Collins can look into the sources of stress in your life and see what ways of reducing or managing those stresses you two can develop. That would help me decide if it will be possible to avoid an increase in medication that I think it would be safer to do without."

Indicators: "Ms. Ruiz was working successfully for quite a while, even though she was coping with headaches. I suspect that if she can get a bit of control, even if it is a small reduction in her frequency or intensity of headaches, she would be able to go back to work. That would make a significant difference for her family financially and would further reduce the stresses she is facing."

In each case, the SSRI statements can be used to gain the acceptance of the patient to the idea of adding a BH clinician to their care and used again in the face-to-face introduction that occurs in the exam room. It is tempting to avoid the difficulties of having the BH clinician on call to the doctor for face-to-face warm handoffs by using the SSRI statements as a way of getting the patient's assent to be scheduled to see the BH clinician at another time. Sometimes this is unavoidable. It is common experience in practice, particularly with patients who sometimes have difficulty keeping appointments, that the face-to-face warm handoffs lead to almost doubling the rate that patients keep subsequent appointments with the BH clinicians as when they are scheduled with the BH clinician without a face-to-face meeting [1].

S: "Ms. Smith is having a very difficult time helping Brandon (3 year old) settle down for bed at night. It is stressing the entire household."

S: "Ms. Johnson is a person with a lot of experience helping parents successfully manage bedtime."

R: "I am hoping that in working with Ms. Johnson you can find a way to reduce the stress of bedtime. Ms. Smith has been having a difficult time managing her diabetes as shown in her very high Hemoglobin A1C (HbA1c) which the stress of bedtime is certainly not helping."

I: "Because if Ms. Smith could get Brandon to bed reliably in under an hour, she could return to exercising in the evening. That would be good for her lipids, her HbA1C, and her peace of mind."

Notice that the aspect of the BH clinician's skill set that is most relevant to the patient's situation is what the doctor stresses. In the case above, Ms. Johnson is a skilled BH generalist, experienced at working with the behavioral health needs of adults and children. But it is not her skills with substance abuse care or depression intervention that make her someone that Ms. Smith would want to work with, it is her skill at making bedtime easier. That is the skill set that is highlighted. In the early stages of their work together, Ms. Johnson will tell Ms. Smith that she is a licensed clinical social worker, but that will be as context to how she learned the techniques or skills she is teaching Ms. Smith. Ms. Smith is not interested in picking the expertise that is being added to the team for her benefit by discipline. The techniques she will learn could be taught by team members from a number of disciplines, licensed and unlicensed. She wants the person who can best help her get her child to sleep.

S: "Bob reports he is experiencing the early stages of a recurrence of his depression."

S: "Mr. Gonzalez has a lot of experience helping people keep minor recurrences of depression from developing into major episodes."

R: "I am hoping that while working with Mr. Gonzalez, you can get back on track fairly quickly. I would like to get an update from the two of you in 3 weeks so that we can reinstitute medication if that is indicated."

I: "Because if Bob is able to get through a mild recurrence of his depression without losing traction in his work or social life, I think it will give him confidence about planning for his future, something that up to now he hasn't quite been able to do."

On paper this may seem like a complex process, but try reading the examples out loud. You get a complete statement that would require less time than is usually taken for either the hall discussion or the in-room introduction.

When it is possible with schedules, it is also effective to have a "report back" to the doctor by the BH clinician and the patient. It orients the doctor briefly to the specifics of what was useful in their work together. It allows the BH clinician to say complimentary things about the patient and sometimes vice versa. It passes the role of clinician regarding behavioral aspects of the patients' care back to the doctor and enfranchises him or her to remind the patient of the skills that they learned in working with the BH clinician when those skills could be useful in the future.

The SSRI conversation can start the practice of discussing patients' situations between team members with the patient participating on a broader basis. It allows for other members of the team to see examples of what such a conversation looks like. It is much easier to have conversations about the care of patients in their presence than most team members can imagine. No one needs to change the facts that are discussed, though it helps to have a change in some of the types of languages in which the facts are couched. Table 6.1 offers some examples of ways that usual professional language, which tends to characterize patients in ways that are either passive or negative or both, can be transformed into characterizations that are active and positive.

As a way to build the skills of team members in having conversations in front of patients that engage and activate patients in their own care, have the team practice, adding to the list in Table 6.1. At first, they are likely to experience the process as humorous and forced. It is not what they "really think" about the patients. If you imagine or role play using these terms in clinical practice, the impact begins to come clear. When the experience of the patient is factored into the exercise, and the difference in the behavior that the patient is likely to exhibit begins to become apparent, people begin to

TABLE 6.1 Examples of ways to change your language to engage and activate your patient

Negative/passive words	**Positive/active words**
Suffers from	Struggles with
Refused to take	Decided against
Did not keep appointment	Was unable to be here
Was noncompliant with	Had not seen the value of
Arrived late	Was determined not to miss

see this as an exercise designed to make their work lives much easier. They begin to feel the descriptions take on more authenticity.

As team members get more comfortable in having conversations in the presence of patients, as their characterizations become more active and positive than they have used in the past, they tend to develop greater comfort and skill at speaking with patients generally. This is not something to force, but it is something worth cultivating or nurturing. Some BH clinicians strengthen this skill by reading back their note from the last time to the patient at the start of each subsequent visit. It is regular practice in saying things briefly and with active and positive characterizations. It is training for the patient to participate in the conceptualization of their care. It is also a way to keep notes simple and clear enough that doctors find them useful and read them regularly as they go in to see the patient.

The discussions of complex or challenging patients in the weekly team meetings, combined with an increase in precision at using language effectively with patients, constitute graduate-level course content in behavioral health practice for the whole team. The facility and comfort of team members at bringing each patient into the conversation about their own needs and treatment become a central skill set that they share. This allows the team to move from endorsing the patient's participation in their own care team as an aspirational idea, to being able to facilitate this process in day-to-day practice. This is one way that a practice might be said to move from good to great in team-based patient-centered primary care.

In many practices in which BH clinicians have been part of the treatment team long enough for the fact of integration not to constitute a new way of working anymore, nonclinical members of the team, such as medical assistants, care managers, and community health workers, have begun to take on carefully delineated areas of behavioral healthcare in the same way that they take on carefully delineated areas of medical care [9]. With the advent of ways for nonclinical team members to take courses toward master's degrees in counseling or social work, your team may become the source for generating your future BH clinicians.

Maintaining the Team

If your team is able to develop as you hope, it can bring a few new challenges. One challenge is that team members who become more skilled and who can operate more independently will at some point want to be compensated for what they are able to do that is not able to be done by other people with the same job title. The fact that their work life is more interesting and enjoyable means a great deal, but eventually you may need some avenues for augmentation of payment to reduce the pressure that comparison with their peers brings. Augmenting team member roles and compensation by having them train new team members are ways to both maintain current team members and replace the ones who decide to take new opportunities.

The process of onboarding BH clinicians or other roles is important and deserves careful attention. The culture that you have developed can begin to fade if attrition is not used as opportunity to reaffirm and pass on the culture you have developed. (Remember the "mission speech"?) Watching other team members work at the beginning of a new team member's tenure can be worth much more in the long run than quickly filling up their schedule to take the load off their colleagues. New team members should watch all of the rest of the team work, not just members in the same job category, if they are to begin to understand and join the culture and practices that you have worked so hard to develop. Pairing them with team members to help them learn the skills as well as the culture of the team is an important investment for the future of the team. The culture that you have spent so much effort building can gradually dissipate through the addition of nonacculturated team members, if the process of onboarding is short-changed.

Summary

In a very few pages, I have tried to go from the basics of adding behavioral health to your practice all the way to refinements that could help you build a truly great primary care health team. This is a process that is ongoing. I believe that, in addition to the evolution of methods and workflows that are occurring in the "exemplar integrated practices," we are seeing changes in the fundamental ways that medical and behavioral problems are defined and understood in these practices. When all of the patients' disorders, stresses, and problems are seen together and in the context of their family, culture, and social situation, new patterns emerge that can help us find new approaches to helping. The disappearing of the bright line between physical and behavioral processes that is has been occurring in research in neurology, endocrinology, immunology, and psychology is being translated into practice in highly evolved integrated primary care settings. While creating new ways of conceptualizing the problems that our patients bring to primary care is not the goal of anyone at the start of the process of behavioral health integration, it keeps the whole endeavor exciting and rewarding well beyond the initial benefits of better access for patients and greater satisfaction for doctors.

References

1. Apostoleris NH, DeGirolamo S, McConarty P, Mazyck B. Overcoming barriers to mental health utilization: examining the referral process in a community health center-based family medicine residency. Poster presented at the conference of the Society of Teachers of Family Medicine. May, 2005.
2. Barkham M, Connell J, Stiles W, Miles J, Margison F, Evens C, Mellor-Clark A. Dose-effect relations and responsive regulation of treatment duration: the good enough level. J Consult Clin Psychol. 2006;74:160–7.
3. Blount A. Integrated primary care: Organizing the evidence. Fam Syst Health. 2003;21:121–34.

4. Dwight-Johnson M, Unutzer J, Sherbourne C, Tang L, Wells KB. Can quality improvement programs for depression in primary care address patient preferences for treatment? Med Care. 2001;39:934–44.
5. Hall J, Cohen DJ, Davis M, Gunn R, Blount A, Pollack DA, Miller WL, Smith C, Valentine N, Miller BF. Preparing the workforce for behavioral health and primary care integration. J Am Board Fam Med. 2015;28:S41–51.
6. Katon W, von Korff M, Lin E, et al. Stepped collaborative care for primary care patients with persistent symptoms of depression: a randomized trial. Arch Gen Psychiatry. 1999;56:1109–15.
7. Kroenke K, Spitzer RL. The PHQ-9: a new depression diagnostic and severity measure. Psychiatr Ann. 2002;32:509–15.
8. Robinson P, Reiter J. Behavioral consultation in primary care. 2nd ed. Geneva, Switzerland: Springer International Publishing; 2016.
9. Roy-Byrne P, Craske MG, Sullivan G, et al. Delivery of evidence-based treatment for multiple anxiety disorder in primary care: a randomized controlled trial. JAMA. 2010;303(19):1921–8.
10. Solberg LI, Crain AL, Maciosek MV, et al. A step-wedge evaluation of an initiative to spread the collaborative care model for depression in primary care. Ann Fam Med. 2015;13:412–20.
11. Thota AB, Sipe TA, Byard GJ, et al. Collaborative care to improve the management of depressive disorders: a community guide systematic review and meta-analysis. Am J Prev Med. 2012;42:525–38.
12. Wagner EH, Austin BT, Davis C, Hindmarsh M, Schaefer J, Bonomi A. Improving chronic illness care: translating evidence into action. Health Aff. 2001;20:64–78.

Chapter 7
Measure What Matters

Deborah J. Cohen and Bijal A. Balasubramanian

Preamble

Clinicians feel professional accountability to evaluate what they do—the scientific side of their disciplines. And as a practical matter, they want to discover how their integrated behavioral health efforts are affecting the practice. Are we making a difference? What difference and to whom? Are the "darts" hitting near the bull's-eye? If not, how can we improve our aim? Measuring is key to improving "aim." But what to start measuring—according to what principles? What evaluation framework can give meaning and coherence to all the specific measurements? Clinical teams do not have to become researchers to use quality improvement methods to learn from experience, improve their "aim," and demonstrate value. *CJP*

D. J. Cohen (✉)
Department of Family Medicine, Oregon Health & Science University, Portland, OR, USA
e-mail: cohendj@ohsu.edu

B. A. Balasubramanian
Department of Epidemiology, Human Genetics, and Environmental Sciences, UTHealth School of Public Health in Dallas, Dallas, TX, USA

Introduction

There is substantial evidence that integrating medical and behavioral healthcare improves healthcare quality, patient experience, and can help reduce healthcare costs [1–5]. In this chapter, we make the case that "measurement"—the act of monitoring and using a standard unit or instrument to assess the degree to which something changes [6]—is a key activity for improving and maintaining quality in your practice, and it is therefore an important aspect of integrating medical and behavioral healthcare for your patients. Measuring is critical in general, but specifically, in the case of integration, measuring allows your practice to assess the quality *of* integrated care you deliver (e.g., do patients' depression symptoms abate?) and your practice's quality *for* integrating care (e.g., are the changes your practice is implementing to integrate care reaching patients that need them?). Measuring is also important to sustain the integrated care changes your practice makes, so that you continually evolve your approach to balance pressures of the external environment and the needs of the patients you serve. These data can also be used to advocate for enhanced payment, which is important for sustainability.

We had the opportunity to lead the evaluation of an integrated care initiative called Advancing Care Together (ACT) [7, 8]. The goal of ACT was to change practice to provide patients with comprehensive, whole person care. Drs. Gold and Green describe this program in Chap. 1. We worked with practices to measure implementation of the integration changes they were making and the quality of care delivered to their patients. We did this by identifying a small number of clinically meaningful measures. These were care processes and outcomes that practices were using as a part of routine clinical care. We developed a way for practices to document this information so that it supported clinical care and could also be used to measure changes in care delivery and changes in care quality. For instance, ACT practices wanted to know how consistently they were assessing patients for depression symptoms with the Patient Health Questionnaire (PHQ)-2 [9], and then if the PHQ-2 was positive, how consistently they were assessing patients with the PHQ-9. Practices generated reports, either using their electronic health record (EHR) system or manually, to measure these screening rates, and looked at these reports regularly to monitor and improve the quality for delivering integrated care (i.e., increasing systematic screening for depression symptoms). While measuring added extra work, practice members were willing to do this for a few reasons. First, the data they agreed to collect would help their practice understand the reach and impact of the changes they were making. Second, these data provided clinical teams with the information they needed to stay informed about status of patients' conditions. If a patient's depression symptoms were not improving, clinical teams wanted to know that and change the treatment approach. Third, the ACT practices wanted the larger clinical community to know that the work that they were doing could change patient outcomes, and it did [10].

It is possible, even likely, that as you start measuring integrated care in your practice that you will experience some challenges in making measuring and monitoring delivery of integrated care a routine aspect of your practice functions. You may feel that your practice lacks the tools and experience needed for measuring. In this chapter, we share a practical way to think about and start measuring integration in your clinic. You can start out small, by identifying and measuring a few key care processes and clinical outcomes that you and your practice feel are meaningful markers of how well your practice is integrating care and the extent to which the changes you are making improve care quality. We identify some important measures of integration to consider, point you to some resources where you can find more measures, and describe a process for measuring that is adaptable and hopefully adoptable for your practice.

Guiding Principles for Measurement

Through our work in ACT, we identified several principles that guide our thinking about measuring. These principles may help you and your practice think about how to approach measuring and how to make this a routine practice activity.

- Measuring is an activity that your practice does to improve and maintain quality. Measuring helps you identify where and when improvements are needed for existing care processes, understand when changes are working (e.g., are improving patient care) or not, and monitor quality to ensure the changes you make are maintained.
- Make measuring a part of everyday practice workflow by choosing clinically meaningful measures that are sensitive to change. This can help make measuring a normal and accepted part of the clinical care process. Consider how these data can inform care team huddles and outreach and how data can be summarized to inform clinical care.
- You cannot measure everything, and not everything should be measured. Measure care processes (e.g., appropriate screening with PHQ-9) that are on the path to changing outcomes (e.g., resolution or reduction of depression symptoms). This will help you understand how well your practice is implementing your integration approach and reaching the patients you target. This will also help you understand why a change you have implemented may or may not change outcomes. Choose outcome measures that are aligned and are good indicators of clinical quality.
- Measuring process and outcomes at the practice, clinician, clinical team, and patient levels is necessary for quality improvement.
- What you measure will—out of necessity—evolve. It is good to review the reasons for measuring certain quality markers so that you know why you are measuring something.

What Clinical Process and Outcomes Should I Be Measuring?

There are a number of good resources to help practices think about evidence-based changes you might want to implement (e.g., assessing patients' level of diabetes distress [11]) as part of integrating care. The Academy: Integrating Behavioral Health and Primary Care is an Agency for Healthcare Research and Quality (AHRQ)-funded website with many resources for practices integrating care. The Atlas of Integrated Behavioral Health Care Quality Measures (https://integrationacademy.ahrq.gov/resources/ibhc-measures-atlas) provides some ideas for measurement. This web resource also includes a "Playbook" for integrating care that includes a section about using data in quality improvement (https://integrationacademy.ahrq.gov/playbook/collect-and-use-data-quality-improvement). In addition, a published paper on integrating psychosocial and medical care for patients with diabetes includes recommendations for clinical assessment, endorsed by the American Diabetes Association, that can be used to measure quality [12].

Table 7.1 reflects what is suggested in some of the resources that we mention earlier. It identifies measures that we have found useful in our work with practices that are integrating care. We offer these as a starting place. Making measuring a routine part of delivering high-quality integrated care takes time and, therefore, requires motivation. Choosing measures that people in your practice are motivated to collect—measures that are meaningful to you and tailored to your practice's needs—is essential.

The measures in Table 7.1 are purposefully selected because they are evidence based and sensitive to change. For example, annual screening for depressive symptoms among patients with a diabetes diagnosis might be a practice quality target. A practice can generate a list of its active adult patients with a diagnosis of type II diabetes mellitus (target population) and calculate the percentage who have a PHQ-2 and/or PHQ-9 in the past year. This percentage would let the practice know if they are meeting their target. At the same time, generating a list of patients with diabetes and routinely checking if patients on that list have been screened and/or screened positive for depression symptoms can also be a strategy to improve care quality, particularly when combined with outreach. This example shows why measuring for quality improvement is best when the measures chosen are aligned with clinical care process and outcomes; it ensures that you are monitoring and improving patient care and quality improvement simultaneously.

TABLE 7.1 Process and outcome measures to consider for measuring quality of integrated care

RE-AIM element [13, 14]	Measures/data collection approach
Reach: The absolute number, proportion, and representativeness of individuals who are willing to participate in a given initiative *Did the integration intervention reach the intended target population?*	*Numerators*: **Level 1**: # target patients screened (e.g., AUDIT, PHQ9, GAD7, chronic illness target) **Level 2**: # of patients screened positive **Level 3**: # of patients screened positive who needed treatment that were treated *Denominator*: All patients in the practice who are in the target population, as defined by practice *Demographic data*: Practice tracked patient age, gender, insurance type, race/ethnicity for the above *Source*: EHR and/or manual tracking
Effectiveness: The impact of the intervention on important outcomes *Did the integration approach we implemented change key outcomes?*	Of the patients who screened positive and received the intervention, clinical change was observed in measures that are tailored to the practice change, including: *Depression symptoms* — measured by PHQ9 [9] *Anxiety symptoms* — measured by GAD7 [15] *Substance use* — measured by AUDIT [16] *Diabetes distress* [11] *Chronic care management* — measured by items such as blood pressure, medication adherence, self-management, HbA1c *Source*: EHR and/or manual tracking

TABLE 7.1 (continued)

RE-AIM element [13, 14]	Measures/data collection approach
Adoption: For practices, these are the number of clinicians and/or clinical teams willing to initiate a program *At what level did clinicians and clinical teams engage and adopt the integrated care approach?*	Per clinician, the percentage of eligible patients that the clinician and his/her team screen and refer to behavioral health clinician and the change in this over time *Source*: EHR data and/or manual tracking; it can also be useful to talk with clinicians and teams to understand barriers/facilitators to engagement
Implementation: The extent to which elements of the intervention approach you develop is done consistently and as intended *What is the fidelity to the integration process and workflow changes you want to make? What elements are adapted and why? What works and what does not and why?*	Your practice will identify key elements of your integration approach. It might be useful to spell out these elements for people in the practice Team leads can observe and talk with staff to ensure that key elements are consistently implemented, and if they are not being done or how they are being done has been modified, team leads can learn why *Source*: While some measures might be tracked, implementation may be best assessed through periodically watching team care, asking team members to be self-aware of processes, asking questions and storytelling
Maintenance: The extent to which the integration changes your practice makes becomes institutionalized or part of the routine organizational practices and policies *Is your practice able to sustain the integrated care changes?*	Talk with practice operation leads to determine how best to sustain integration changes your practice makes, if they improve care outcomes Keep measuring key processes and outcomes to ensure that changes you and your practice made are maintained

Clinical teams will likely not adopt and implement these integration changes uniformly. Measuring process and outcomes that are tied to clinical quality can foster adoption and also help you identify teams within your practice that are excelling at the change. Having those team members share their experiences with others can promote adoption and spread of integration within your practice.

Next, we offer a practical framework for how you and your practices can approach measuring integrated care quality.

A Framework for Measuring Integration in Your Practice: RE-AIM

You will notice that the measures in Table 7.1 are aligned with Reach, Effectiveness, Adoption, Implementation, and Maintenance or RE-AIM [13, 14]. This is a practice-friendly framework for thinking about measuring and monitoring clinical quality. We often use the RE-AIM framework in our research because it is a simple and pragmatic way of thinking about measuring [17, 18]. We found this to be true for measuring integration in ACT [19]. There are other approaches that can also be applied to measuring and monitoring clinical quality in practice; Getting to Outcomes (GTO) is another widely used framework your practice may find useful [20].

Reach helps identify if the people who should have received an intervention/service did receive it. Reach requires defining the target population intended for your integration program (e.g., all patients with a diagnosis of type II diabetes). It is best to include only those patients to whom your practice can feasibly provide integrated services. Reach tells us to assess the following: Of this target population, how many people received the intervention/service as intended? Reach is the proportion of patients in the target population (denominator) who received the intervention/service (numerator). It is useful to consider measuring Reach at multiple levels. For example, you might screen all of your patients with type II diabetes for depression with a PHQ-2. Level 1 Reach is the proportion of patients with type II diabetes that received a brief screen for depression symptoms. Of those patients that screen positive, your approach might then be to screen those patients with a PHQ-9. Level 2 Reach, therefore, is the proportion of patients with type II diabetes screened positive with the PHQ-2 (denominator) that were administered a PHQ-9 assessment (numerator). Of those that screen positive on the PHQ-9 (denominator), your practice might have a treatment approach that involves, perhaps, a conversation with a clinician (who might determine everything is okay) and/or a warm handoff to a behavioral health clinician (BHC) (numerator). Level 3 Reach would be the proportion of patients who screened positive on the PHQ-9 that were then touched by a primary care and/or behavioral health clinician. As this example suggests, each step in the process involves counting the number of people that should have received screening or treatment. Assessing Reach will push your practice to clarify the details of the care process and path for patients with, for instance, diabetes. Measuring Reach can help identify barriers to implementing a new care process. For example, if you are measuring Reach, you will know if too few patients are being screened for depression. Perhaps there is a problem with the workflow that you can identify and address. Measuring Reach can help your practice continuously refine the change process until it is systematized into usual care [19].

The "E" in RE-AIM is Effectiveness. Effectiveness reminds us to measure the effect of implementing integrated care on patients' health outcomes. This could be a decrease in depression symptoms [10], lower blood pressure, and hemoglobin AIC values, as well as shorter-term changes, such as improvements in diet and exercise.

Adoption helps you assess and understand who in your practice has (or has not) embraced the integrated care changes that you planned and worked to implement. Adoption is an important indicator of spread of the intervention, and tracking Adoption can help encourage uptake of integration innovation practice-wide.

Studying Implementation helps to refine the steps your practice takes to implement integration to increase Reach and maximize Effectiveness. This includes the processes or steps you go through to make these changes, why some changes are implemented and some are not, as well as why some changes in clinical process did or did not lead to better integration and better outcomes. Awareness and assessment of issues related to implementation are important for practices that are integrating care. For instance, a practice might start to integrate care for its patients by hiring a new professional to help deliver behavioral healthcare to patients. We call these professionals behavioral health clinicians (BHCs). It is common that in a few weeks after hiring a BHC the practice finds this person is fully booked [21]. The practice had hoped that the BHCs would be available for warm handoffs, what we define as impromptu BHC visits with patients during a scheduled medical encounter. Understanding why the BHC is unavailable is likely a question of practice and process changes, or in other words implementation. Consider finding answers to questions such as the following:

- How long are the BHC visits?
- How are BHC visits scheduled? [21]
- How complex are the patients who have been referred to the BHC?
- What resources does the BHC have to refer patients with more complex needs? [22]
- Where is the BHC located? [23] Is this person nearby and visible?
- How does the primary care clinician or medical assistant find the BHC when he or she is needed?
- What are your practice's rules for interrupting the BHC when he or she is with a patient? [24]

All of these factors, and others, contribute to explaining why the BHC may not be available for warm handoffs, which can be a crucial integration implementation challenge. Methods that are more qualitative in nature, such as observing workflows around planned integration changes and process mapping by practice coaches/facilitators, are a great way to identify and understand integration implementation challenges and to gather the information needed to address these challenges. (Also see Chap. 4 for suggestions on how to prevent this common pitfall from occurring.) A primary care clinician or BHC that is aware of and observes his or her own processes or behaviors will be able to identify and talk about what is and is not working with regard to implementing integration. Additionally, the stories that people in the practice share with each other can help identify changes that are needed to achieve the process and outcome goals you set for integration.

In research and in practice, we often want to know if the changes practices implement to improve care quality are maintained. Once you have reached a point of stability with the implementation of integrated care, continuing to measure and review critical clinical markers of integration is important to maintaining quality of care, and measuring markers for integration is important to ensuring that the changes your team implemented are maintained. This allows you to know when a quality marker slips so you can take steps to bring it back to goal.

How Do We Get Started?

Here are some steps that we think might help you get started. These steps are designed for thinking through how to implement integration in a target population, rather than practice-wide. We did this because many practices just starting out often do not have the resources to implement integration practice-wide. Practices with more experience integrating care or those implementing integration practice-wide may choose to skip the first two steps.

First, use data to identify care gaps. Overall, where is your practice's quality of care strongest and where do you find it needs improvement? You may notice from patient outcome data that a subgroup of patients has poor hypertension control and are not meeting care targets. The first step is reviewing data to identify care gaps. Measuring makes quality gaps visible and addressable. You cannot fix what you cannot see.

There may be multiple care gaps identified. Therefore, a second important step is prioritization. What are the quality gaps that you want to focus on improving and which might be improved by integrating care? This will help you determine the target population that should receive integrated care. It is quite common for practices to want to focus their integration changes more narrowly at first to manage resources and maintain quality. For instance, a practice may make the transition to an integration approach slowly by hiring one BHC. The practice knows this is not enough staff to meet all of practice's patients' needs for integrated care, but it is what the practice can currently afford. In this case, it is important to narrow the target population. Perhaps the target population is patients with hypertension, as mentioned earlier, or patients who are identified as high risk for hospitalization. This definition of the target population will guide both what and how you measure. For example, the target population will now be your denominator for calculating Reach and assessing impact. It will also be the population by which you measure care quality.

Next, clearly describe the practice changes you will be implementing to integrate care. This step entails identifying all process of care changes and describing what each process entails, including which patients are targeted, the steps in the process, who does each step, and what is documented. One way to do this is with flow diagrams. We have included an example of a flow diagram in Fig. 7.1. These diagrams help you and your team understand the care changes that need to be made and what roles and workflows these changes affect. For example, your practice might switch from an approach to identifying patient depression that relied on clinician discretion to one that uses systematic, periodic screening with an assessment tool. What your practice is adding to the care process is screening. The practice may decide that the first step in screening will be accomplished by the front-desk staff handing patients a paper screener (PHQ-2). The medical assistant will review the results and determine if it is positive. If the PHQ-2 is positive, the medical assistant is tasked with administering the PHQ-9, noting both scores in a template in the electronic health record (EHR) and mentioning this to

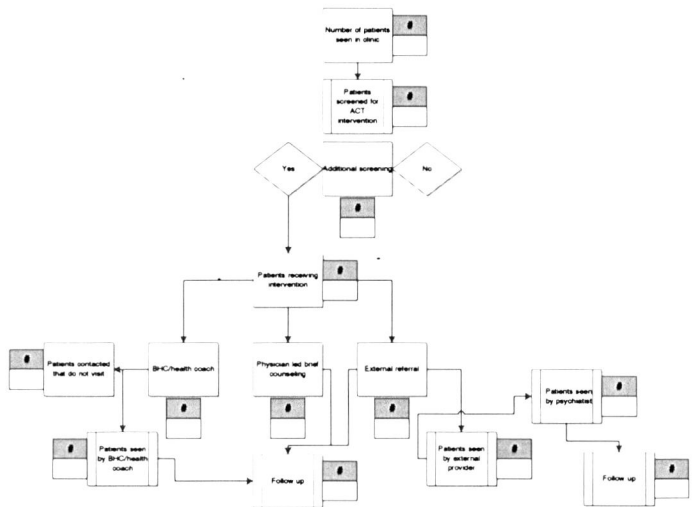

FIGURE 7.1 Example of an intervention process diagram

the clinician before he or she enters the examination room with the patient. Given this change, you might want to measure rates of this new screening process to assess adoption and implementation of these changes.

The fourth step is to engage practice members in measuring. It is important that the people delivering patient care have input into and support the measures selected. Their work is likely being evaluated through the measuring process, and including them in the decision-making process about what to measure is vital. We recommend including a broad representation of practice staff across roles, as this fosters practice-wide buy-in [25, 26]. There will need to be a person leading this process, who reviews the literature—if necessary—and is knowledgeable about the measures your practice is already held accountable for by external agencies. You will want to align with those. This lead person will provide the others in the practice with information about measures and develop a process for making measurement decisions.

Your practice will also need to establish a process for measuring. Here, aligning measuring with care delivery can reduce real and perceived burden that can be associated with measurement. This is true whether the EHR is used to generate data for measuring or if this needs to be done manually. Ideally, the data you use for measuring would be routine information the clinician or clinical team member would need to document anyway as part of delivering good clinical care. It is possible that your EHR will lack the functionality needed to support both delivery and measurement of integrated care [27]. Consider working with a vendor or an expert to tailor your EHR to meet your practices' documentation and measurement needs. If this is not possible and your EHR is not a good tool for documenting and extracting clinical data for purposes of measurement, we have included some very simple tracking tools in Figs. 7.2 and 7.3 that we developed. These tools can be adapted to help you track basic information about the patient care you deliver so this information can later be tabulated for quality measurement.

Conclusion

"If you don't measure it, you can't improve it." We heard this aphorism echoed by practice staff at a recent quality improvement meeting we attended. This practice has been doing quality improvement for a long time, and they know how important measuring is for implementing change and for knowing if changes are impacting care quality. Starting small, measuring clinically meaningful process and care quality markers, and aligning measuring with clinical care delivery for integration are a few of the principles we cover in this chapter that will make measurement seem more accomplishable and help your practice start using data to guide improvement in practice process and care quality.

The measurement approach we describe here is meant to align with your quality improvement process and provide your practice a clinically relevant and realistic way to evaluate the changes you make in your practice. This approach translates the methods we use in our scientifically rigorous

Chapter 7 Measure What Matters   171

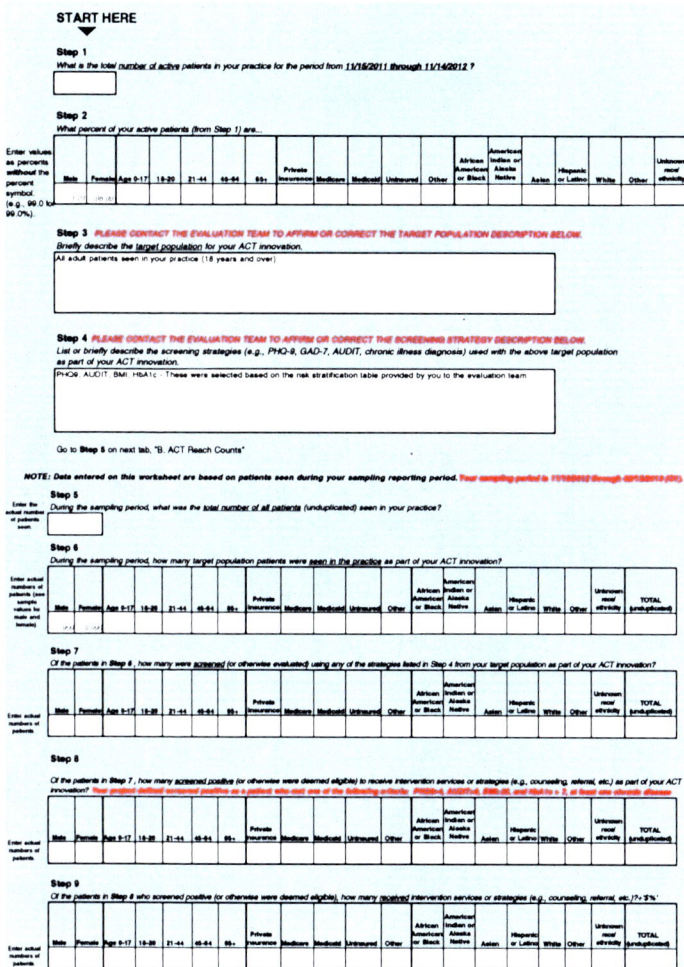

FIGURE 7.2 ACT reach reporter

evaluations for use in the practice setting. The principles, measures, and steps we describe can be used to facilitate measuring, continuous learning, and quality improvement in your practice. This can ensure the integrated approach you implement (and all of the practice changes you make) are maintained at the highest quality.

Dummy ID	Medical Record Number	Date of Visit	Date of Screening	Screen positive		Referral?			Intensive counselling?				Follow up?
Please use the correct dummy ID for patients who screened positive	This column is for your internal use. Please maintain a copy of this file with this number. Please do not send files with medical record numbers or patient names.	Please provide the date of this visit	Please provide date patient was most recently screened on or prior to date of visit (Column C)	What behavioral test did patient screen positive for? 1=PHQ9>4 2=AUDIT>8 3=Both 4=don't know	What medical test did patient screen positive for? 1=HbA1c>7 2=HbA1c>7 3=Both 4=don't know	If this patient's screen was "positive" did the patient receive a referral? 1=Yes 2=No 3=Don't know	If this patient's screen was "positive" did the patient receive a referral? 1=Yes 2=No 3=Don't know	If this patient's screen was "positive" did the patient receive a staff referral? 1=Yes 2=No 3=Don't know	If referred, did patient receive intensive counseling from primary care? 1=Yes 2=No 3=Don't know	If referred, did patient receive intensive counseling from BHC? 1=Yes 2=No 3=Don't know	If referred, did patient receive intensive counseling from HC? 1=Yes 2=No 3=Don't know	If referred, did patient receive intensive counseling from referral? 1=Yes 2=No 3=Don't know	If referred, was patient followed-up? 1=Feedback from psychiatry 2=Feedback from HC/BHC 3=No show 4=Don't know
		9/5/2013	8/28/2013	1	4	2	2	2	1	3	2	2	2	4
		9/19/2013	8/21/2013	1	4	2	2	2	1	3	2	2	1	2
		9/26/2013	9/20/2013	4	4	2	2	2	1	3	2	2	1	2
		9/26/2013	9/24/2013	1	4	2	2	2	1	3	2	2	1	2
		10/24/2013	10/15/2013	4	4	2	2	2	1	3	2	2	1	2
		10/24/2013	10/7/2013	1	4	2	2	2	1	1	2	2	1	2
		11/8/2013	10/17/2013	1	4	2	2	2	1	1	2	2	1	2
		11/11/2013	10/30/2013	4	4	2	2	2	1	3	×	2	1	2
		11/11/2013	11/18/2013	4	4	2	2	2	1	1	2	2	1	2
		11/12/2013	11/4/2013	4	4	2	2	2	2	3	2	1		2

FIGURE 7.3 Example of a patient tracking sheet

References

1. Butler M, Kane RL, McAlpin D, et al. Integration of mental health/substance abuse and primary care no. 173. Rockville, MD: Agency for Healthcare Research and Quality; 2008.
2. Katon WJ, Unutzer J. Health reform and the Affordable Care Act: the importance of mental health treatment to achieving the triple aim. J Psychosom Res. 2013;74(6):533–7.
3. Collins C, Hewson DL, Munger R, Wade T. Evolving models of behavioral health integration in primary care. In: Milbank Memorial Fund report; 2010.
4. Unutzer J, Katon WJ, Fan MY, et al. Long-term cost effects of collaborative care for late-life depression. Am J Manag Care. 2008;14(2):95–100.
5. Gallo JJ, Zubritsky C, Maxwell J, et al. Primary care clinicians evaluate integrated and referral models of behavioral health care for older adults: results from a multisite effectiveness trial (PRISM-e). Ann Fam Med. 2004;2(4):305–9.
6. OED Online. 2017. http://www.oed.com/viewdictionaryentry/Entry/11125
7. Davis M, Balasubramanian BA, Waller E, Miller BF, Green LA, Cohen DJ. Integrating behavioral and physical health care in the real world: early lessons from advancing care together. J Am Board Fam Med. 2013;26(5):588–602.
8. University of Colorado Department of Family Medicine. Advancing care together. http://www.advancingcaretogether.org/. Updated 2018.
9. Kroenke K, Spitzer RL, Williams JB. The PHQ-9: validity of a brief depression severity measure. J Gen Intern Med. 2001;16(9):606–13.
10. Balasubramanian BA, Cohen DJ, Jetelina KK, et al. Outcomes of integrated behavioral health with primary care. J Am Board Fam Med. 2017;30(2):130–9.
11. Fisher L, Glasgow RE, Mullan JT, Skaff MM, Polonsky WH. Development of a brief diabetes distress screening instrument. Ann Fam Med. 2008;6(3):246–52.
12. Young-Hyman D, de Groot M, Hill-Briggs F, Gonzalez JS, Hood K, Peyrot M. Psychosocial care for people with diabetes: a position statement of the American Diabetes Association. Diabetes Care. 2016;39(12):2126–40.
13. RE-AIM – Reach Effectiveness Adoption Implementation Maintenance. 2017. www.reaim.org.

14. Glasgow RE, Vogt TM, Boles SM. Evaluating the public health impact of health promotion interventions: the RE-AIM framework. Am J Public Health. 1999;89(9):1322–7.
15. Spitzer RL, Kroenke K, Williams JB, Lowe B. A brief measure for assessing generalized anxiety disorder: the GAD-7. Arch Intern Med. 2006;166(10):1092–7.
16. Saunders JB, Aasland OG, Babor TF, de la Fuente JR, Grant M. Development of the Alcohol Use Disorders Identification Test (AUDIT): WHO collaborative project on early detection of persons with harmful alcohol consumption—II. Addiction. 1993;88(6):791–804.
17. Balasubramanian BA, Cohen DJ, Davis MM, et al. Learning evaluation: blending quality improvement and implementation research methods to study healthcare innovations. Implement Sci. 2015;10:31.
18. Cohen DJ, Balasubramanian BA, Isaacson NF, Clark EC, Etz RS, Crabtree BF. Coordination of health behavior counseling in primary care. Ann Fam Med. 2011;9(5):406–15.
19. Balasubramanian BA, Fernald D, Dickinson LM, et al. REACH of interventions integrating primary care and behavioral health. J Am Board Fam Med. 2015;28(Suppl 1):S73–85.
20. Wandersman A, Alia K, Cook BS, Hsu LL, Ramaswamy R. Evidence-based interventions are necessary but not sufficient for achieving outcomes in each setting in a complex world: empowerment evaluation, getting to outcomes, and demonstrating accountability. Am J Eval. 2016;37(4):544–61.
21. Davis MM, Balasubramanian BA, Cifuentes M, et al. Clinician staffing, scheduling, and engagement strategies among primary care practices delivering integrated care. J Am Board Fam Med. 2015;28(Suppl 1):S32–40.
22. Cohen DJ, Balasubramanian BA, Davis M, et al. Understanding care integration from the ground up: five organizing constructs that shape integrated practices. J Am Board Fam Med. 2015;28(Suppl 1):S7–20.
23. Gunn R, Davis MM, Hall J, et al. Designing clinical space for the delivery of integrated behavioral health and primary care. J Am Board Fam Med. 2015;28(Suppl 1):S52–62.
24. Cohen DJ, Davis M, Balasubramanian BA, et al. Integrating behavioral health and primary care: consulting, coordinating and collaborating among professionals. J Am Board Fam Med. 2015;28(Suppl 1):S21–31.

25. Bleser WK, Miller-Day M, Naughton D, Bricker PL, Cronholm PF, Gabbay RA. Strategies for achieving whole-practice engagement and buy-in to the patient-centered medical home. Ann Fam Med. 2014;12(1):37–45.
26. Nutting PA, Crabtree BF, Miller WL, Stewart EE, Stange KC, Jaen CR. Journey to the patient-centered medical home: a qualitative analysis of the experiences of practices in the National Demonstration Project. Ann Fam Med. 2010;8(Suppl 1): S45–56; s92.
27. Cifuentes M, Davis M, Fernald D, Gunn R, Dickinson P, Cohen DJ. Electronic health record challenges, workarounds, and solutions observed in practices integrating behavioral health and primary care. J Am Board Fam Med. 2015;28(Suppl 1):S63–72.

Chapter 8
Where Practice Meets Policy

Stephanie R. Kirchner, Stephanie B. Gold, and Benjamin F. Miller

Preamble

The larger business and policy environment can affect what is easier or harder to do in the practice, where to find moral or tangible support, and what battles to pick or where to step back and do workarounds. Understanding the business and policy environment can help guide your actions and load your innovation for success. This does not mean that clinicians need to become policy wonks. Policy development is often local—where clinicians live and work. Your own work can inform policy if you think of it as having policy significance—and bring it forward. You can influence policy as a clinician who is looking forward to fewer workarounds that result from delayed policy change. *CJP*

S. R. Kirchner (✉) · S. B. Gold
Eugene S. Farley, Jr. Health Policy Center, Aurora, CO, USA

Department of Family Medicine, University of Colorado School of Medicine, Aurora, CO, USA
e-mail: stephanie.kirchner@ucdenver.edu

B. F. Miller
Well Being Trust, Oakland, CA, USA

© Springer Nature Switzerland AG 2019
S. B. Gold, L. A. Green (eds.), *Integrated Behavioral Health in Primary Care*, https://doi.org/10.1007/978-3-319-98587-9_8

Introduction

Transforming primary care practices to integrate behavioral health, bringing together historically separated physical and behavioral health, is a dramatic undertaking — in large part because of the underlying policies that have separated payment, training, and information sharing between these two fields of patient care. This chapter outlines some of the barriers and solutions associated with financing integrated care in your practice, workforce constraints, and data and information sharing. It also introduces ways that you as a primary care leader can influence the healthcare delivery system to move toward more integrated, whole-person care. Specific payment models, workforce training opportunities, and privacy laws in the United States are described. Dealing with policy issues is always a local affair, and details here may not be applicable to other countries; however, in many instances, health policy challenges and their solutions are universal. We place particular emphasis on financing and payment, as it is essential in accomplishing sustainable integrated care and must be addressed at some level to be successful. The overarching message of this chapter is that it is critical to understand the context that you are working within so that you can determine what you may need to accept or work around to move toward your integration goals and what you can influence moving forward.

Payment

Most current payment mechanisms reimburse delivery of specific services rather than providing prospective funds, and many artificially separate physical and behavioral health benefits. Fractured payment makes it difficult to sustain a primary care practice with integrated behavioral health clinicians [1, 2]. Various payment models have been tested in integrated settings, each demonstrating pros and cons in supporting integrated care [3, 4] (Table 8.1).

TABLE 8.1 Pros and cons of existing payment models for integrated behavioral health

Payment model	Description	Pros	Cons
Fee-for-service	Provides retrospective reimbursement based on certain billing codes for specific, individual services to patients	• Incentivizes productivity in terms of volume of services • Some opportunity to create and make available codes for specific integrated services	• No incentives for efficient care or limiting unnecessary care • Limited reimbursement for non-face-to-face services; reimbursement for redesigned services has to be added to billing codes piecemeal • Often limitations on what type of clinician (social worker, psychologist, other therapist) can use certain codes • Some states or payers may not allow billing codes for physical and behavioral health services on the same day

(continued)

TABLE 8.1 (continued)

Payment model	Description	Pros	Cons
Blended fee-for-service and capitation (fee-for-service plus PMPMs for care coordination, case management, or PCMH services)	Provides prospective payment for non-face-to-face services or services not billable under fee-for-service; may be specific to certain care components (e.g., care coordination)	Prospective payment increases flexibility in how, where, and by whom care is provided	• PMPM amount may be insufficient to cover non-face-to-face services or consumed by nonbehavioral health needs • Fee-for-service as the underlying model continues to overemphasize volume of services; same limitations as above

TABLE 8.1 (continued)

Payment model	Description	Pros	Cons
Pay for performance (P4P)	Provides reimbursement for achieving defined and measurable goals related to care process and outcomes, patient experience, utilization patterns, or cost targets	Can improve care quality, efficiency, accountability, and coordination when appropriate measures are selected and agreed upon	• Difficult to operationalize and measure outcomes • Poorly accounts for complexity when providing care for multiple conditions • May not align with patient preferences • May incentivize "cherry picking" low-risk, compliant patients and firing high-risk, noncompliant patients • Burden in data collection and reporting may detract from patient care

(continued)

TABLE 8.1 (continued)

Payment model	Description	Pros	Cons
Bundled (episode of care) payments	Provide single reimbursement for a group of services related to a treatment or condition that can involve multiple providers in multiple settings	• May increase coordination between multiple providers • Supports flexibility and how and where care is delivered • Incentivizes efficient management of a healthcare episode • Simplifies billing • Holds providers accountable for a single episode of care	• Difficult to separate care for a patient with multimorbid conditions into primary care bundles (i.e., what would belong in diabetes vs. depression bundle) • May limit patient choice in providers or location of care • No incentive to limit future episodes • May incentivize "cherry picking" low-risk, compliant patients and firing high-risk, noncompliant patients

TABLE 8.1 (continued)

Payment model	Description	Pros	Cons
Shared savings	Provide bonus payment for having total cost of care below a predetermined benchmark, contingent on also meeting set quality targets. Accountable Care Organizations paid via PMPM amounts; practices may still be paid fee-for-service	• Creates an incentive to decrease costs • Links ability to receive savings to meeting quality targets • Incentivizes coordination across settings if done at the level of an ACO	• When providers or practices still reimbursed on a fee-for-service basis, they receive conflicting incentives • May incentivize "cherry picking" low-risk, compliant patients and firing high-risk, noncompliant patients if risk adjustment is not done properly • Determination of risk-adjusted PMPMs requires sophisticated data modeling

(continued)

TABLE 8.1 (continued)

Payment model	Description	Pros	Cons
Global capitation (with risk adjustment)	Provides a single risk-adjusted payment for full range of healthcare service needs of a specific population for a fixed period of time	• Supports flexibility in care delivery • Simplifies billing • Incentivizes efficient and coordinated care • Incentivizes collaboration with other providers for a particular patient population • Emphasizes preventive services and overall health	• Determination of risk-adjusted PMPMs requires sophisticated data modeling • May decrease patient choice • May incentivize "cherry picking" low-risk, compliant patients and firing high-risk, noncompliant patients if risk adjustment is not done properly • Potential for services to be withheld (inappropriate under-delivery of services) • Potential for PMPM amount to be consumed by nonbehavioral health services

Fee-for-service provides retroactive reimbursement based on certain billing codes for specific, individual services to patients [5]. Fee-for-service fundamentally supports volume over value and because it is dependent upon billing codes, it limits the types of services reimbursed when delivered by an integrated behavioral health clinician. Though billing codes have been added by some payers (see list below) to reflect billing options for integrated behavioral health, they do not always encompass the full spectrum of services behavioral health clinicians provide in the primary care setting. Additionally, some states or payers may limit the ability for billing for physical and behavioral health services on the same day or not recognize services delivered by certain types of behavioral health clinicians. This model of payment also lends itself to increased clinician burnout rates as providers are financially incentivized to see as many patients as they can in as short a time possible [6].

Blended fee-for-service and capitation includes payments for care coordination, case management, or other patient-centered medical home (PCMH) services through an additional per-member, per-month (PMPM) amount on top of fee-for-service to cover non-face-to-face services.

Pay for performance (P4P) provides additional payment for meeting certain outcomes or improving on a measure and can be added to either fee-for-service or capitation. The success of this model depends on what outcomes or process measures are selected and how they are incentivized. Most P4P metrics are disease oriented rather than whole person oriented (e.g., blood sugar control for a patient with diabetes vs. their health-related quality of life) and emphasize process rather than outcome measures (e.g., checking urine microalbumin for a patient with diabetes rather than decreased incidence of diabetic nephropathy).

Bundled payments reimburse for a discrete set of related treatments or an "episode" of care in a lump sum rather than paying individually for each clinical interaction or service. Bundled payment can be difficult to operationalize in primary care because of the complexity around what constitutes an episode of care.

Shared savings allow practices or an overarching organization to share in savings with a payer if their costs are less than a predetermined benchmark and quality targets are met. This model has been primarily operationalized in the United States through Accountable Care Organizations (ACOs), which are groups that agree to work together to share accountability for costs and outcomes and may include health plans, hospitals, provider organizations, and others. ACOs are paid through a PMPM amount, though reimbursement is often still done on a fee-for-service basis at the level of the practice.

Global payment/capitation pays a predetermined per person rate to practices, regardless of the delivered services [4]. With prospective budgeting, global payment allows the practice to determine who the right professionals are to have on the team to meet the needs of their specific patient panel. Concerns about inadequate funds for higher-needs patients can be addressed through risk- adjusting the PMPM amounts.

Any model that is based on upfront payment simplifies billing and supports flexibility in care delivery; rather than requiring continual additions of billing codes to support integrated services and changes in care redesign, a single amount can be applied to patient care as practices see fit. At the same time, upfront payment also runs the risk of incentivizing the exclusion of sicker patients if funds are not sufficient; appropriate risk adjustment of these amounts is key. There is also a risk of funds being used up by physical health needs in places where the value of investing in integrated behavioral health may not have been recognized and there are no other incentives for coordinating physical and behavioral healthcare.

In addition to giving prospective payments in the form of a PMPM, an upfront lump sum can be given specifically calculated for the costs of integrating behavioral health. In one evaluation this payment mechanism was found to lead to cost savings for public payers (e.g., Medicaid) primarily through a reduction in utilization [7].

While global or other prospective payments may be the most promising solutions to this problem, there are ways to support on-site behavioral health services in the current fee-for-service model. While not ideal, as they still promote a separate service line for behavioral health, these mechanisms help financially support a practice working toward increased access to behavioral health services for patients and families. Same-day billing for physical and behavioral health services must be allowed by the payer to use these codes on the same day as a physical health visit. The behavioral health clinician billing the services must also be a recognized provider type by the payer; for certain codes only psychologists or psychologists and licensed clinical social workers may be able to bill. Codes for traditional psychotherapy may be used, and some primary care practices have been able to partially or even fully support their integrated services through billing of their behavioral health clinician's time in this manner. There are a variety of time-based Current Procedural Terminology (CPT) codes for individual, family, and group psychotherapy; commonly used codes include 90832 for 16–37 min of individual psychotherapy, 90834 for 38–52 min of individual psychotherapy, and 90846 and 90847 for 26 min or longer of family psychotherapy without and with the patient present, respectively.

These codes for traditional psychotherapy, however, do not apply to many integrated services. Additional codes have been created by some US payers to account for other behavioral health services in primary care:

1. Health and Behavior Assessment and Intervention codes: These codes apply to services for patients who may not necessarily have a mental health diagnosis or a mental health diagnosis that is central to intervention. These 9600 series CPT codes require a physical health diagnosis but can be used by behavioral health clinicians when they address an assortment of behavioral health needs related to physical health issues, including

patient adherence to medical treatment, symptom management, health-promoting behaviors, health-related risk-taking behaviors, and overall adjustment to physical illness.
2. Collaborative Care codes: Beginning in 2017, the Centers for Medicare and Medicaid Services (CMS) approved payment for behavioral health services for patients participating in a Collaborative Care Model program through Current Procedural Terminology (CPT) codes 99492, 99493, and 99494. These programs join psychiatrists and care managers trained in behavioral health with primary care clinicians to systematically manage and monitor a panel of patients with behavioral health issues in the primary care setting [8].
3. General Behavioral Health Integration code: CMS created an additional code in 2017, CPT code 99484, for integrated services that do not fall under the Collaborative Care Model but do include elements such as systematic assessment and monitoring, facilitation of behavioral health treatment, and care plan revision for patients who are not improving. This code does not require a psychiatrist and/or a behavioral healthcare manager [8].

Other nonbilling alternatives to consider include seeking out grant funding to build your initial infrastructure and considering where you could receive in-kind support from mental health centers or other community organizations and resources. Research your local philanthropic organizations to see if this work would be in line with their mission.

With knowledge in hand of the above mechanisms to pay for integrated behavioral health, there are a few basic questions that a primary care practice may wish to ask to better understand payment models offered from their own individual payer mix (Table 8.2). This checklist of questions will help your practice understand the payment context in which you practice and arm you to leverage data in making a business case for alternative payment.

TABLE 8.2 Questions to ask to understand your financial situation and prepare a business case for integration

What is the payer mix for your patients? (What percentage of your practice's patients are self-pay, Medicaid, Medicare, and private insurance? What are the percentages across different private plans?)

What details in your payer contracts are relevant to providing integrated services? (If you have not already done so, familiarize yourself with your payer contracts.)

Which payers allow same-day billing of physical and behavioral health services?

For each major payer, what types of behavioral health clinicians are able to bill for services in primary care? [9]

What alternative payment models are available through each major payer? What are the requirements for participation?

Do all of your payers allow billing of Health Behavior Assessment and Intervention codes, Collaborative Care Model codes, and General Behavioral Health Integration codes?

Does your practice have a prospective budget that includes estimated costs of behavioral health services? (Do not limit your estimated costs to clinician salary. Consider training, possible workspace reconfiguration, overhead costs, and staff time spent on tasks related to supporting integration.)

Based on your current or planned approach to integrate behavioral health, what utilization, cost, and quality benefits can be modeled based on prior research or your current practice data? (Consider which conditions may show the greatest potential for cost savings. Melek et al. provide useful modeling to support your case [10].)

What are the financial impacts of your decisions on patients? (For example, will the patient have to pay a separate co-pay to see the on-site behavioral health clinician?)

This checklist exercise will lead to greater understanding of your situation and where you may be able to take advantage of current opportunities and optimize billing practices. The exercise may also bring to light significant gaps in your ability to finance integrated services and help set an agenda for negotiating with payers and how you may wish to get involved with advocating for improved payment for integration on a broader scale (Table 8.3). Having answered the questions above, the next step is to meet with payers to share your laid-out vision for enhanced care that contains costs and improves quality and the resources you need to make that care possible.

TABLE 8.3 Workarounds and policy change opportunities for integrated behavioral health: payment

Working within current constraints	• Examine your current payment situation using the above checklist, including establishing a prospective budget for integration • Maximize use of available fee-for-service codes • Seek out grant funding for start-up costs • Bring your business case to payers to advocate for alternative payment models more supportive of integrated behavioral health
Opportunities for policy change (i.e., what to ask of policymakers)	• Eliminate carve-outs of behavioral health services • Allow for same-day billing of physical and behavioral health services where fee-for-service is still the predominant payment method • Use risk-adjusted global budgets or other prospective payment methodologies to fund comprehensive primary care services • Include in global payment models specific incentives for inclusion of behavioral health services

Workforce

Even if no challenges related to payment for integrated services existed, inadequate numbers and geographic maldistribution of primary care-trained behavioral health clinicians can create barriers to integrating care. These workforce challenges are magnified when looking for behavioral health clinicians who focus on children and teens. Practices starting out on their integrated care journey have found it difficult to find behavioral health clinicians with experience or training in integrated settings and frequently underestimate the time it takes for retraining to adapt traditional mental health training to primary care [11].

Depending on the type of integrated care approach used, patient needs, and payment opportunities, partnering with behavioral health clinicians of different roles and training backgrounds may make more sense for your practice. Roles employed for integrated behavioral health services may include counselors or therapists, care managers, social workers, and psychiatric consultants, as in the Collaborative Care Model described above in Chap. 6. Other roles are emerging that support behavioral health services and bridge to social health, such as community health workers, regional health connectors, and peer support specialists. Counseling or therapy is conducted by Licensed Clinical Social Workers (LCSWs), psychologists, addiction counselors, and licensed marriage and family therapists or other master's-level counselors. Behavioral healthcare managers may have any of these educational backgrounds or may be registered nurses with additional behavioral health training. Consultation for medication management is done by psychiatrists, psychiatric advanced practice providers (psychiatric nurse practitioners or physician assistants), or clinical pharmacists. The educational background for community health workers, regional health connectors, and peer support specialists is variable; peer support specialists generally will have personal experience with behavioral health issues [12].

Developing a behavioral health clinician training program can grow the future workforce in your area; growing on your own is possible and may be the most efficient way to proceed if your local resources are not adequate. Pioneering organizations in behavioral health integration, like Cherokee Health Systems (https://www.cherokeehealth.com/professional-training/) and Salud Family Health Centers (https://www.saludclinic.org/fellowships), trained their own behavioral health clinicians and now support training the workforce for other practices. As an example of diverse ways to be involved in workforce training, Cherokee Health Systems offer practicum experience to social work and psychology students, accredited psychology internships, postdoctoral fellowships, and Integrated Care Training Academy conferences to share best practices with other organizations [13].

Other resources exist to support retraining of behavioral health clinicians and necessary training of other clinic providers and staff. University of Massachusetts' Primary Care Behavioral Health certificate program (https://www.umassmed.edu/cipc/pcbh/overview/) provides advanced training through online courses for behavioral health clinicians to work in integrated settings. Practice Transformation Organizations and other groups providing technical assistance related to integration can support the training that needs to occur across all clinicians and staff to understand how best to function as an integrated team.

In Chaps. 3 and 4, Scott Hammond and Caitlin Barba describe their use of external partnerships with outside behavioral health organizations as an alternative to internal hiring that redistributes the existing behavioral health workforce to provide services in primary care. As with hiring a behavioral health clinician internally who has not worked or trained in integrated settings, additional training and onboarding will likely be necessary when pursuing an external partnership.

Rural communities face additional challenges with workforce recruitment and retention, and in these areas stigma often prevents patients from seeking community resources where behavioral health services are traditionally located. This highlights some of the benefits of access to integrated services; patients receive whole-person care in one location where they are most accustomed to accessing healthcare.

In spite of workforce shortages, behavioral health staffing needs can also be met through alternative solutions in rural areas. Telehealth connects behavioral health clinicians from other locations to a practice without local resources. This can include service provision in real time, such as through telehealth counseling, or as in the case of the Extension for Community Healthcare Outcomes (ECHO) model, through case-based learning and consultation separate from patient visits. Psychiatry consultation for medication management can occur within or outside of patient visits. In the United States, there are CMS billing codes for telehealth services that occur in real time with the patient present [14]. Sharing behavioral health clinicians across practice sites is another possible solution. These workarounds to meet workforce needs are summarized in Table 8.4 along with opportunities for broader-scale policy change.

TABLE 8.4 Workarounds and policy change opportunities for integrated behavioral health: workforce

Working within current constraints	• Consider creating a behavioral health clinician training program to "grow your own" • Hire behavioral health clinicians with integrated care experience or, if not available, take advantage of available integrated training programs or technical assistance • In rural areas, use telehealth to bring behavioral health services to your patients where they are not otherwise available
Opportunities for policy change (i.e., what to ask of policymakers)	• Develop a workforce assessment strategy including what data elements will be assessed, how it will be reported, and what entity will be responsible for setting and meeting goals [15] • Fund programs for scholarships or loan repayment for behavioral health clinicians in underserved areas • Create fee-for-service billing codes for telehealth services that do not occur in real time with the patient present

Privacy and Information Sharing

Regulations and policies related to patient privacy and data sharing vary in different countries. Though usually designed to protect patients, they may limit how personal health information is protected and shared between care providers. Understanding the nuances of these protective measures may help clinicians more effectively coordinate patient care across providers (Table 8.5).

There are two primary pieces of federal legislation and regulation affecting information sharing related to behavioral health diagnoses in the United States: the Health Insurance Portability and Accountability Act of 1996 (HIPAA) and 42 Code of Federal Regulations Part 2 (42 CFR Part 2), most recently updated in 2017. The good news is that both HIPAA and 42 CFR Part 2 do not apply to internal communication; for integrated practices, providers on the same team taking care of the same patient do not need a written disclosure to share information. These rules are relevant for bidirectional information sharing with external organizations, however,

TABLE 8.5 Workarounds and policy change opportunities for integrated behavioral health: information sharing

Working within current constraints	• Familiarize yourself with local privacy laws in addition to federal/national laws • Update your patient consent and authorization forms with information regarding sharing behavioral health information across team members; consider adapting existing consent forms and/or consulting legal counsel
Opportunities for policy change (i.e., what to ask of policymakers)	• Eliminate requirements under 42 CFR Part 2 in the United States or other laws to obtain written patient consent for each disclosure of PHI when for the purposes of treatment, payment, or healthcare operations

which is important when coordinating patient care with other entities such as specialty behavioral health.

HIPAA applies to any general disclosure of protected health information (PHI). For most types of health information, this generally does not create barriers to information sharing, because there are exceptions for disclosure without authorization for the purpose of treatment, payment, or healthcare operations (including care management and quality improvement), as long as the patient has received notice of the practice's privacy policy. However, these exceptions do not apply to psychotherapy notes (these notes document conversations with patients in individual or group settings that are kept separately from information about diagnosis and treatment and the rest of the medical record); sharing these requires specific written authorization [16].

42 CFR Part 2 protects any information disclosed by a covered program that identifies an individual directly or indirectly as having a current or past drug or alcohol problem or as a participant in a covered program. Covered programs include those that: (1) are federally certified or supported through federal tax exemption or federal funding and (2) "holds itself out as providing, and provides, substance use disorder diagnosis, treatment, or referral to treatment" [17]. This is commonly understood to refer to specially licensed substance use treatment facilities such as methadone clinics; there has been confusion regarding where this applies to general medical facilities such as primary care practices. Unless related to a medical emergency or mandatory reporting, 42 CFR Part 2 requires written patient consent for each disclosure of PHI, even for the purposes of treatment, payment, or healthcare operations [18]. There are specific requirements for disclosure authorization forms, including listing what information will be shared. Within a primary care practice, a provider may be subject to this regulation if they are part of an identified unit within the clinic that meets the criteria above or their "primary function" is substance use disorder diagnosis, treatment, or referral. If a

primary care clinician provides screening, brief intervention, or referral to treatment as a part of general medical care, this does not meet the definition of a Part 2 program. Primary care clinicians waivered to prescribe buprenorphine are not "categorically included" but may be subject to these regulations on a case-by-case basis. If it is unclear if your practice falls under these regulations, legal counsel and guidance may be appropriate [19].

Some states and jurisdictions have additional privacy laws; it is important to familiarize yourself with any other information-sharing restrictions that apply to your integrated efforts. Once you have familiarized yourself with the appropriate laws and regulations, revise your general patient consent and authorization forms to include sharing of behavioral health information within the care team. Some local organizations may have standardized consent forms you can use or adapt.

The Larger Policy Context

Enhanced support for integrated care is in sight. With increasing recognition that primary care practices will manage much of their patients' behavioral health needs, more and more policies and programs are laying the groundwork for primary care practices to integrate [20].

Different countries have different laws affecting integrated care. Such laws can be complicated and create quite a web of rules and regulations. There have been a number of laws in the United States supporting parity of behavioral health insurance coverage with physical health coverage, including the Mental Health Parity Act of 1996, Medicare Improvements for Patients and Providers Act of 2008, Mental Health Parity and Addiction Equity Act of 2008, and components of the Patient Protection and Affordable Care Act of 2010. For health plans that offer both physical and behavioral health services, these laws combined require that behavioral health services are covered at least as favorably as physical health services, including any specific lifetime or annual dollar limits, annual visit limits, copayments, and deductibles. The Affordable Care Act includes behavioral health as one of the Essential Health Benefits, which means that for any health plans on the marketplace or in individual or small-group markets, both physical and behavioral health services must be covered.

The Medicare Access and CHIP Reauthorization Act (MACRA) of 2015 created two pathways for payment that shift away from purely fee-for-service reimbursement, the Merit-based Incentive Payment System (MIPS) and advanced Alternative Payment Models (APMs). Every practice that sees more than 100 Medicare patients or charges more than $30,000 a year in services to Medicare must participate in one of these payment pathways. Practices that do not see at least 20% of their Medicare patients in an advanced APM or receive at least 25% of Medicare payments through an advanced APM are automatically enrolled in MIPS.

MIPS adjusts Medicare reimbursements up or down depending on performance in quality, cost, practice improvement activities, and advancing care information (use of electronic health records). The practice improvement activities include a subcategory for behavioral health integration, so integrated practices will find their work recognized by the point system. APMs employ payments apart from fee-for-service that can be used flexibly in primary care, which may provide opportunity for supporting integration even if it is not a specific component of the program. One APM, the Comprehensive Primary Care Plus Initiative, includes a requirement for integrating behavioral health for its advanced practices. Over time, more opportunities for participating in APMs will become available.

International Policy

Outside of the United States, integrated behavioral health has been implemented successfully across countries with a range of economic and political circumstances, including those with models of health insurance that are employer-based, a national health system, or a regulated individual market. The United

Kingdom, Japan, and the Netherlands provide examples of national movements toward integrated behavioral health under varying models of health insurance. In the United Kingdom, which has a national health system, success of a program based in the Collaborative Care Model called Improving Access to Psychological Therapy led to a national investment in expansion. This program includes P4P incentives based on improvement on symptom measures. Similarly in the Netherlands, which has a regulated individual market, the Collaborative Care Model has been adopted nationwide. Behavioral health services are included in essential benefits of insurance packages. In Japan, which has mixed employer-based and government-run insurance, all prefectures in the country are required to assess and respond to behavioral health needs as part of a comprehensive healthcare plan [21].

The challenges faced across these countries echo those of the United States, with needs for: changing culture through strong leadership and shared values on whole-person care, development of new models of interdisciplinary training, strengthening and connecting health information technology between primary care and behavioral health clinicians, enhancing flexibility of payment models and accounting for start-up costs, and capability to assess benefits in different sectors such as unemployment or disability [21].

Sufficient primary care infrastructure is a necessary precondition for integrated care, which may be lacking in low- and middle-income countries. Lessons learned from these settings include the need for ongoing support of primary care workers, availability of psychotropic medications, and strong linkages to higher levels of care and community resources [22].

Interested in Doing More?

In each of the sections above on payment, workforce, and information sharing, we have concluded with not only ways to work within current constraints but also suggestions for broader policy change. There is a much-needed role for primary care leaders to have a voice in advancing such policy change for integrated behavioral health and a variety of ways to do so.

1. Share your story widely

Combining patient stories and data can be an impactful tool when advocating for change, not only with payers but also with other stakeholders, including policymakers and the public. Practices may find themselves in the position to testify, present their work, or speak to media on what they are doing and what may need to be done to help their patients. Speaking out to a larger group of stakeholders can help advance broader scale change by demonstrating the benefits of integrated behavioral health.

2. Consider involvement in demonstration projects to support transforming your practice and also inform future changes in policy

Participating in pilot opportunities and Centers for Medicaid and Medicare Innovation projects, such as State Innovation Model initiatives and the Comprehensive Primary Care Plus initiative, is a proactive step to both receive support for practice transformation at the forefront of change and inform future policy and payment models through data collection and reporting to federal partners. Though they often involve an investment of time and practice resources, most provide technical assistance and some provide alternative payment to test innovative approaches to provide patient care, including behavioral health integration.

3. Join groups or multi-stakeholder efforts in a position to influence healthcare delivery

Find out who is responsible for making decisions locally and what groups are advocating for similar goals. Such groups may include professional organizations (i.e., local chapters of physicians or behavioral health clinician organizations), issue-specific organizations (i.e., advocacy groups focused on behavioral health conditions), and project-specific organizations (i.e., stakeholder groups related to practice transformation demonstrations). Allocating resources and time to participate in multi-stakeholder meetings provides the opportunity to share both what is working and what is not in your community. It also creates awareness of what services exist in a community and highlights gaps, both increasing leverage between existing partners and eliminating redundancy in efforts. Participating gives you a forum to learn from others and collectively inform and/or implement policy.

Conclusion

Redesigning your practice to provide integrated care is a journey that requires coping with your current policy environment, particularly with regard to payment, workforce, and information sharing. Practices that navigate these policy issues find they do not ever want to return to the old way of doing things. Fortunately, policies are changing to make doing the right thing easier and maintain integrated care in your practice, and those who are inclined to do so can support driving these changes forward.

References

1. Kathol RG, Butler M, McAlpine DD, Kane RL. Barriers to physical and mental condition integrated service delivery. Psychosom Med. 2010;72(6):511–8.
2. Kathol RG, deGruy F, Rollman BL. Value-based financially sustainable behavioral health components in patient-centered medical homes. Ann Fam Med. 2014;12(2):172–5.
3. Hubley SH, Miller BF. Implications of healthcare payment reform for clinical psychologists in medical settings. J Clin Psychol Med Settings. 2016;23(1):3–10.
4. Miller BF, Ross KM, Davis MM, Melek SP, Kathol R, Gordon P. Payment reform in the patient-centered medical home: enabling and sustaining integrated behavioral health care. Am Psychol. 2017;72(1):55–68.

5. Hussey PS, Ridgely MS, Rosenthal MB. The PROMETHEUS bundled payment experiment: slow start shows problems in implementing new payment models. Health Aff. 2011;30(11):2116–24.
6. Reck J. Primary care provider burnout: implications for states and strategies for mitigation. National Academy for State Health Policy. 2017. https://nashp.org/wp-content/uploads/2017/01/VCU-Burnout.pdf.
7. Ross KM, Gilchrist EC, Melek SP, Gordon PD, Ruland SL, Miller BF. Cost savings associated with an alternative payment model for integrating behavioral health in primary care. Transl Behav Med. 2018:iby054. https://doi.org/10.1093/tbm/iby054
8. Medicare Learning Network. Behavioral health integration services. MLN Factsheet. Centers for Medicare & Medicaid Services. January 2018.
9. National Conference of State Legislatures. Mental health benefits: state laws mandating or regulating. 2015. http://www.ncsl.org/research/health/mental-health-benefits-state-mandates.aspx.
10. Melek SP, Norris DT, Paulus J, Matthews K, Weaver A, Davenport S. Potential economic impact of integrated medical-behavioral healthcare: updated projections for 2017. Milliman Research Report. January 2018.
11. Hall J, Cohen DJ, Davis M, Gunn R, Blount A, Pollack DA, et al. Preparing the workforce for behavioral health and primary care integration. J Am Board Fam Med. 2015;28:S41–51.
12. Skillman SM, Snyder CR, Frogner BK, Patterson DG. The behavioral health workforce needed for integration with primary care: information for health workforce planning. Center for Health Workforce Studies, University of Washington. 2016.
13. Cherokee Health Systems. Professional training. 2018. https://www.cherokeehealth.com/professional-training/. Accessed 8 Mar 2018.
14. Medicare Learning Network. Telehealth services. MLN Factsheet. Centers for Medicare & Medicaid Services. February 2018.
15. Block R. Behavioral health integration and workforce development. Milbank Memorial Fund Issue Brief. May 2018.
16. Office for Civil Rights. HIPAA privacy rule and sharing information related to mental health. United States Department of Health and Human Services. 2014.
17. Department of Health and Human Services. Confidentiality of substance use disorder patient records. 42 CFR Part 2. Fed Regist. 2017;82(11):6052–127.

18. Integrated Behavioral Health Partners. Federal framework for sharing behavioral health information. 2018. http://www.ibh-partners.org/get-started/behavioral-health-data-sharing-toolkit/legal-issues/#federalframework
19. Freeman DS, Hudgins C, Hornberger J. Legislative and policy developments and imperatives for advancing the Primary Care Behavioral Health (PCBH) model. J Clin Psychol Med Settings. 2018;25(2):210–23.
20. Zivin K, Miller BF, Finke B, et al. Behavioral health and the Comprehensive Primary Care (CPC) initiative: findings from the 2014 CPC behavioral health survey. BMC Health Serv Res. 2017;17(1):612.
21. Pincus HA, Jun M, Franx G, van der Feltz-Cornelis C, Ito H, Mossialos E. How can we link general medical and behavioral health care? International models for practice and policy. Psychiatr Serv. 2015;66:775–7.
22. Funk M, Ivbijaro G. Integrating mental health into primary care: a global perspective. Geneva & London: World Health Organization & WONCA; 2008.

Chapter 9
Closing: It Is a Journey, Not a Destination

Larry A. Green and Stephanie B. Gold

Preamble

If successful, this book has provided "maps" and practical wisdom for moving forward with integrated behavioral health (BH) — more of a journey than specific a destination. This closing chapter reprises this guidance from the book's authors, who represent broad expertise in integrating care. If you keep moving along this path, incorporating these pioneers' lessons learned from experience, the benefits will accrue and your practice will become more of what you probably always wanted it to be. *CJP*

Introduction

Your journey to integrated primary care and behavioral health (BH) will be unique, while at the same time being similar in some ways to practices that have paved the way

---

L. A. Green (✉) · S. B. Gold
Eugene S. Farley, Jr. Health Policy Center, Aurora, CO, USA

Department of Family Medicine, University of Colorado School of Medicine, Aurora, CO, USA
e-mail: larry.green@ucdenver.edu

pioneering integrated care such as Westminster Medical Clinic. You can now proceed knowing quite a lot about what you are getting into, aware of the realities faced by other primary care practices daring to disrupt themselves to be better. You can be enabled by evidence from research and practical experience from the frontlines of healthcare. You can join what has become a professional movement toward care that replaces a line between behavioral and physical health with a better, integrated approach that treats patients more comprehensively, as whole persons.

You know that integrated care is a well-developed, well-thought-out, important change in primary care practice. It is not a crazy idea attractive to a few idealists out of touch with what real practice is all about. Indeed, the evidence is irrefutable; it can be done, even in less than ideal situations. The substantial changes that integrated care entails will require adaptive leadership from you and your entire practice, teamwork that delivers new services in revised workflows, and acquiring and using data to guide your journey. Your local policy situation will probably constrain your efforts in some ways, perhaps requiring some adaptive workarounds but also offering you a further chance to advocate for rules and regulations that enable your new, integrated care.

It is likely that you will find your own voice as you explain what integrated care is, why you are disrupting your practice to achieve it, and how you are going about it. You can probably accelerate your progress by being intentional in how you lead, develop your team, acquire and use data to guide your work, and tend your local policy environment. If you wish you can anchor your work in the advice from colleagues presented as Fig. 1.2 and put it on a wall in your practice as a reminder of what you are doing and how you are doing it:

1. Integrated care is not a minor adjustment but a paradigm shift we need to make toward patient-centered, whole-person care.
2. It is important that we prepare ourselves for this transformation and define relationships and protocols upfront, understanding they will evolve.

3. It will take all of us as an inclusive, empowered team to get this done, with everyone taking on leadership responsibilities.
4. We will learn as we go, adjusting to our mistakes, engaging our patients early and often, welcoming help from each other and from outside our practice.
5. We will collect and use data that matter to us to measure our progress, be accountable to ourselves, and to show others what we are accomplishing.

The ideas and suggestions in this book are intentionally specific to integrating primary care and behavioral health, but you may find them to be relevant to other substantial changes you may want to make in your practice. They are consistent with the science of diffusion of innovations and how innovations in healthcare are implemented successfully [1]. The rate of adoption of innovations within an organization, such as integrated care in your practice, depends upon how your practice perceives integrated care and its benefits, its compatibility with your shared values, and your collective ability to simplify what can be simplified in your approach. Of course, your progress will also depend on personal characteristics of you and your team—such as your comfort levels with change. And you must do this in the real world of the practice, system, and community you live and work in, which may be wildly enthusiastic about integrated care or hesitant to move forward.

To re-enforce the guidance offered by each chapter's authors, let us reprise some of the key messages of this book.

Reprise of Key Messages

From Chap. 2, What Is Integrated Behavioral Health?:
Integrated behavioral health is:

> The care that results from a practice team of primary care and behavioral health clinicians, working together with patients and families, using a systematic and cost-effective approach to provide

patient-centered care for a defined population. This care may address mental health and substance use conditions, health behaviors (including their contribution to chronic medical illnesses), life stressors and crises, stress-related physical symptoms, and ineffective patterns of healthcare utilization [2].

You can and will need to customize this official definition to share with others what it means to you and your practice. For example, to other clinicians and practice staff you might lean on Table 2.4 and say:

"We are expanding our clinic team to do better (and feel better) with the behavioral health dimension of our practice...things our patients already bring with them...that we may not always have the time or experience to do as well as we want."

From Chaps. 3 and 4, A Real-Life Story of Getting Started:

Your vision of integrated care is a "mini-vision" within your practice's overall vision, and every practice has the potential for integrated care when your vision meets determination.

"Remember, change doesn't happen just because it is a good idea."

Recognize that your current business model may not finance integrated care adequately, so be explicit at the outset about what your approach is likely to cost your practice, how you will cover those costs, and your risk tolerance. But do not forget these noneconomic gains of integrated care:

- More meaningful experience among medical and behavioral health clinicians and personal fulfillment by offering collaborative, accessible care to patients. Clinicians enjoy more efficient workflow through timely access to behavioral health.
- Stronger practice culture and staff who want to be engaged as part of solutions resulting in less burnout and lower turnover of team members.
- Enhanced reputation for whole-person, community-based care that attracts new patients.
- Increased patient satisfaction.

Medical and behavioral healthcare have developed into distinct cultures; merging these cultures can prove the most challenging aspect of transformation and requires attention to language and communication. Consider standardizing how you document and share information between primary care and behavioral health clinicians, perhaps using the ADAPT approach:

- Assessment
- Decision-making, logic, and rationale
- Advice for the patient
- Plan for further care
- Tasks, who is responsible for next steps

Your approach may benefit from relationships with external organizations. Explicit, written agreements, such as Westminster Medical Clinic's "Compact," can promote collaboration and avoid misunderstandings (see Appendix A).

The "80/20 Rule" may help determine if a policy or workflow passes muster. Implement policies that apply to at least 80% of patients—but also work as a team to develop solutions for the remaining 20%.

Researching and utilizing available tools and models to plan your journey, including many referenced in these chapters, will save you time and strife down the road. By necessity, this plan must detail how you will conduct staff development and patient engagement.

From Chap. 5, Everyone Leads:

Leadership is not a role for one person but a function shared by all practice members. It is a form of vigilance and fidelity. It sets a vision and a mission, builds teams, supports a productive practice culture, and cultivates the gifts of each individual in the practice.

Your practice is not a machine. It is actually a living organism with key features of living things: a purpose, the ability to sense, and the ability to respond. Treat it accordingly as you implement your approach to integrated care, setting the purpose, sensing what is happening, and responding to developments as you go.

Remember that nothing ever works in the real world like it does on paper.

During your journey to integrated care, leaders will emerge from everywhere in your practice.

Celebrate every success and embrace every failure as just "incomplete adjustment."

Put things on the walls of your practice, such as:

- Remember why we are here: to help people become a little healthier.
- Expect problems. Welcome them as a sign that we are alive.
- Speak up. Speak the truth and have no fear.
- Be kind. Kindness trumps cleverness every time.
- Try something, anything, and then fine-tune it. Life is a beta test.
- Bite off more than you can chew. Then offer—*offer*—some of it to your neighbor.
- You are the best person to do certain jobs. Do those jobs. Do what nobody but you can do.
- Never stop thinking about how to do it better.

It helps for those who are leading the journey to integrated care to be able to say, clearly and succinctly, *what* you are doing, *why* you are doing it, and *how* you are doing it. This can be your "elevator speech," and this chapter concludes with possible answers to all three of these questions that you can adapt to your situation and use repeatedly.

From Chap. 6, It Takes a Team:

One of the first outcomes of a behavioral health clinician joining a medical practice as a team member is that clinician satisfaction goes up. It feels good to share the load.

In the Primary Care Behavioral Health (PCBH) model of integration, the behavioral health clinician becomes part of the infrastructure of the practice, involved in patient care for whatever seems needed at the time.

Having a behavioral health clinician on the team may be the first time a physician is asking a team member for clinical input, not just assistance.

Chapter 9 Closing: It Is a Journey, Not a Destination

Remember that teams do not just spring into existence and the nature of your team will vary according to the approach you take to integrated care, as illustrated in this chapter. Be intentional and pay attention to:

- Who you hire (Remember also the eight questions to consider asking in an interview tucked into Chap. 4)
- How they are deployed into the practice
- Building a collaborative team culture
- Communication within the team and with patients
- Revisions in workflows
- Maintaining your team

All primary care practices have opinions about meetings, and you will need to decide how and when meetings are needed. Barely having enough time for any meetings can lead to barely enough communication to keep things moving and enjoy the advantages of teamwork and the resulting integrated care. Perhaps the most useful regular meeting is the huddle just before each session of patient care.

Remember to consider using the mnemonic of SSRI to organize the passing of a patient's relationship with a primary care clinician to a behavioral health clinician. It is designed to help doctors know how to conduct this process smoothly and efficiently.

- The first S is for **Situation.** The doctor says to the patient and the behavioral health clinician what *situation* in the patient's current care makes him or her want to add the behavioral health clinician to the treatment team.
- The second S is **Skill Set**. The doctor describes to the patient the *skill set* (as opposed to the discipline) of the BH clinician that makes him the person that he or she wants to add to the treatment team.
- The R stands for **Relationship**. At this point the doctor says what *relationship* the work between the behavioral health clinician and the patient will have to the overall treatment that he or she has been directing. Remember, this is not a new treatment; it is a new aspect of the patient's current care.

- The final I is for **Indicators**. The doctor says to the behavioral health clinician and the patient what would *indicate* that the addition of the behavioral health clinician's expertise and intervention had been successful.

From Chap. 7, Measure What Matters:

Measurement of both processes and outcomes is a necessity to implement, adopt, and sustain integrated care. Your measurement system can empower your entire team. But you do not need to measure everything.

You do need to measure things that will let you understand the impact your approach to integrated care is having on your practice and your patients, stay informed about your patients' conditions, and whether or not you are achieving your goals. Over time, your measurements will help you know what it took for you and your team to integrate care.

You can get started developing your measurement plan by identifying new steps in patient care or gaps in care that you want to close. Define and draw diagrams of workflows showing who does what, when, and where. Constructing such diagrams can anchor what you want to measure to particular points in the path you are taking to improve the care of your patients. Engage the entire team in developing and activating your measurement plan. Responding together to what you learn can be motivating and a lot of fun.

Take care to select measures that can change, i.e., be sensitive to the changes you are making in your practice, e.g., the percentage of patients systematically screened for anxiety and depression. Less can be more and help you not exceed the resources you can devote to measurement. Confirm in advance what your health record system is capable of providing from data already routinely collected and whether or not additional costs are involved.

The RE-AIM framework explained in this chapter is not the only evaluation framework that you could use, but it has been used to good effect by many practices implementing important practice changes. It can help everyone on the team stay on track, understand what is and is not working, identify moments to celebrate, and sustain buy-in to make and sustain the next adaptive change.

From Chap. 8, Where Practice Meets Policy:

This chapter exposes how integrating primary care and behavioral health is still ahead of many policies that were developed for "the old world" and not fully sufficient for the new way of practicing that you are implementing, though the tide is starting to turn.

Regardless of your situation, you will want to pay attention to the payment policies that affect your practice, the availability of the primary care and behavioral health workforce in your community, and access to the clinical and business data and information you need to implement your approach to integrated care.

When your local policies and procedures have not yet caught up with you, unleash your imagination on temporary workarounds and proceed apace.

Conclusion

Robust primary care is probably healthcare's most complex challenge. After all, all health problems exist, sooner or later in primary care settings, and primary care by definition accepts any person of any age or background as a patient. Unavoidably, improving primary care is and always will be an ambitious undertaking. And, wanting to deliver better care tomorrow than today will always be an ambition and duty of primary care clinicians. The tension between what primary care desires to do and what it can do under real-world conditions is real and can be intimidating.

The purpose of this book is now obvious. It aims to go beyond admonitions to integrate behavioral health and primary care as a major practice transformation to gather and share practical knowledge from real, frontline practices that have taken and are still taking the journey to integrated care. It is not a journey for the faint-hearted, nor is it an impossible quest. It is now clear that it can be done and that pioneering successes can be replicated on a wider scale. Indeed, pioneering successes have paved the way for integrated behavioral health to be a global movement. Whole-person care is no longer simply the case in a few bright spots—though these bright spots exist and continue to shine—at places like Cherokee Health Systems in Tennessee, Salud Family Health Centers in Colorado, or the University of Washington that have made integrated behavioral health an inseparable part of primary care.

Integration is starting to be recognized, supported, and rewarded by policymakers and healthcare organizations. In the United States, the National Committee for Quality Assurance (NCQA) now awards Behavioral Health Distinction for patient-centered medical homes that have integrated care and meet certain specifications. The Centers for Medicaid and Medicare Services (CMS) include behavioral health integration as an option for primary care practices to earn points to be reimbursed based on their performance. In several other developed countries, behavioral health integration has been adopted on a national scale. While we are not yet close to optimized systems that enable whole-person care, broader change to support the movement of integrated behavioral health is already in motion.

Why might you decide to initiate your own journey to integrated care now, before optimal systems to support you are in place, when there remains more to learn, policies to change, data problems to solve, and workforce development to do? If you are like most primary care clinicians, you are who you are, doing what you do because you care about people and your community. You do not strive to be mediocre. You strive for excellence and want to improve your practice because it will matter to your patients. Integrated care is not a minor tweak to primary care practice. It is instead a very large, powerful opportunity to make a leap forward to the benefit of not just a few but almost all primary care patients. Our patients are waiting now for healthcare systems in general and primary care in particular to recognize that the mind and body are not separate and must be treated as one. They are waiting to be taken care of the way they see themselves, as whole people. They are waiting to have a reliable place to go with any health problem and receive most of the care they need. They are probably waiting for you to ask them to join your team as expert consultants at every step of your journey.

Maybe something in this book is worth your taking with you on your journey. Please take care of yourself when you join this movement to integrated care and share with your colleagues what you learn as you go. Take heart in knowing that the primary care practices that have already taken the journey do not want to go back to how they used to practice. It is just better care.

References

1. Berwick DM. Disseminating innovations in healthcare. JAMA. 2003;289:1969–75.
2. Peek CJ, National Integration Academy Council. Lexicon for behavioral health and primary care integration: concepts and definitions developed by expert consensus. 2013. http://integrationacademy.ahrq.gov/lexicon.

Appendix A

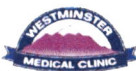 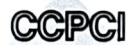 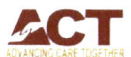

Colorado Center for Primary Care Innovation

Primary Care—Behavioral Health Collaborative Compact

Transition of Care
Mutual Agreement
<ul><li>Maintain accurate and up-to-date clinical records.</li><li>When available and clinically practical, agree to standardized demographic and clinical information format such as the Continuity of Care Record [CCR] or Continuity of Care Document [CCD].</li><li>**Ensure safe and timely transfer of care of a prepared patient*.**</li></ul>

Expectations	
Primary Care	Behavioral Health Care
☐ PCP maintains complete and up-to-date clinical records. ☐ Transfers information as outlined in Patient Transition Record in a timely fashion. ☐ Orders appropriate studies that would facilitate the specialty visit. ☐ Provides patient with specialist contact information and expected time frame for appointment. ☐ Informs patient of need, purpose (specific question), expectations, and goals of the BHP visit. ☐ **Obtains confidentiality release from patient to discuss care with BHP in accordance with federal and state privacy laws*.** ☐ Ensures that patient/family is in agreement with referral, type of referral, and selection of specialist.	☐ Appropriate staff determine and/or confirm insurance eligibility. ☐ **Identifies a specific referral contact person to communicate with the PCMH/PCP*.** ☐ When PCP is uncertain of appropriate laboratory testing, advise PCP prior to the BHP/CP appointment regarding appropriate pre-referral workup. ☐ Informs patient of need, purpose, expectations, and goals of hospitalization or other transfers. ☐ Notifies referring provider of inappropriate referrals and explains rationale.

© Springer Nature Switzerland AG 2019
S. B. Gold, L. A. Green (eds.), *Integrated Behavioral Health in Primary Care*, https://doi.org/10.1007/978-3-319-98587-9

Additional agreements/edits: _____

_____

_____

_____

Access

Mutual Agreement
• **Be readily available for urgent help to both the physician and patient*.** • **Provide adequate visit availability*** • Be prepared to respond to urgencies. • Offer reasonably convenient office facilities and hours of operation. • Provide alternate backup when unavailable for urgent matters. • When available and clinically practical, provide a secure email option for communication with established patients and/or providers.

Expectations	
Primary Care	Behavioral Health Care
☐ Communicate with patients who "no-show" to BHPs and address issues. ☐ **Determines reasonable time frame for BHP appointment*.** ☐ Establishes policy and protocol to facilitate direct communication by phone, email, and in-person with the BHP and patient.	☐ Notifies PCP of first-visit "no-shows" or other actions that place patient in jeopardy. ☐ Schedule patient's first routine appointment with requested provider. ☐ Provides PCP with list of BHPs who agree to compact principles. ☐ Establishes policy and protocol to facilitate direct communication by phone, email, and in-person with the PCP.

Additional agreements/edits: _____

_____

_____

Collaborative Care Management

Mutual Agreement

- **Define responsibilities between PCP, BHP, and patient and identify care team*.**
- **Define PCP and BHP scope of practice*.**
- Clarify who is responsible for specific elements of care (drug therapy, referral management, diagnostic testing, care teams, patient calls, patient education, monitoring, and follow-up).
- Maintain competency and skills within scope of work and standard of care.
- Give and accept respectful feedback when expectations, guidelines, or standards of care are not met.
- Openly discuss and agree on type of care that best fits the patient's needs.

Expectations

Primary Care	Behavioral Health Care
☐ Follows the principles of the Patient-Centered Medical Home or Medical Home Index.	☐ Reviews information sent by PCP and addresses provider and patient concerns.
☐ **Manages the medical or behavioral problem to the extent of the PCP's scope of practice, abilities, and skills*.**	☐ Confers with PCP or establishes other protocol before ordering additional services outside practice guidelines. Obtains proper prior authorization.
☐ Provides designated care coordinator to work with care team, as well as the designated care manager.	☐ Confers with PCP before referring to secondary/tertiary specialists and, when appropriate, uses a preferred list to refer when problems are outside PCP scope of care. Obtains proper prior authorization.
☐ Follows standard practice guidelines or performs therapeutic trial of therapy prior to referral, when appropriate, following evidence-based guidelines.	☐ **Sends periodic written, electronic, or verbal reports to PCP as outlined in the Transition of Care Record*.**
☐ Resumes care of patient as outlined by the BHP, assumes responsibility, and incorporates care plan recommendations into the overall care of the patient.	☐ Notifies the PCP office or designated personnel of major interventions, emergency care, or hospitalizations.
☐ **Shares data with the BHP in timely manner including pertinent consultations or care plans from other care providers*.**	☐ Prescribes pharmaceutical therapy in line with scope of license and insurance formulary with preference to generics, if appropriate to patient needs.
	☐ Provides useful and necessary education/guidelines/protocols to PCP.

Additional agreements/edits: _____

_____

Patient Communication

Mutual Agreement

- Consider patient/family choices in care management, diagnostic testing, and treatment plan.
- Provide to and obtain confidentiality release from patient according to community standards (see Transition of Care).
- Explores patient issues on quality of life in regard to their specific condition and shares this information with the care team.

Expectations

Primary Care	Behavioral Health Care
☐ Explains, clarifies, and secures mutual agreement with patient on recommended care plan. ☐ Assists patient in identifying their treatment goals. ☐ Engages patient in the Medical Home concept. Identifies whom the patient wishes to be included in their care team and participates with team. ☐ **Be available to discuss patient's questions or concerns regarding the consultation or their care management*.**	☐ Informs patient of diagnosis, prognosis, and follow-up recommendations. ☐ Provides educational material and resources to patient when appropriate. ☐ Recommends appropriate follow-up with PCP. ☐ Be available to discuss patient's questions or concerns regarding the consultation or their care management. ☐ **Participates with patient care team*.**

Additional agreements/edits: _____

Appendix B

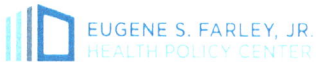

CORE COMPETENCIES
for Behavioral Health Providers
Working in Primary Care

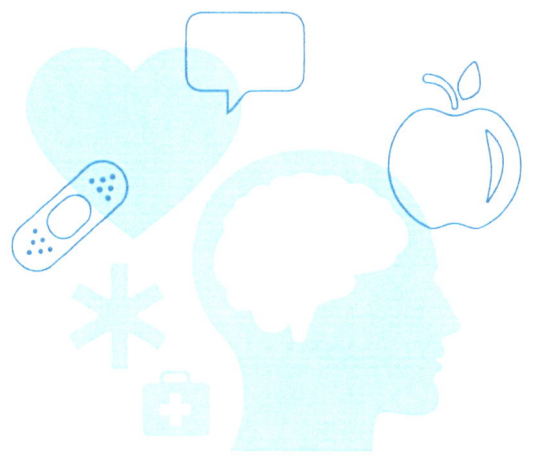

 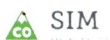 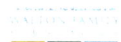 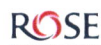

Appendix B

Core Competencies for Behavioral Health Providers Working in Primary Care

This document is in the public domain and may be used and reprinted without permission except those copyrighted materials that are clearly noted in the document. Further reproduction of those copyrighted materials is prohibited without the specific permission of copyright holders.

Suggested Citation

Benjamin F. Miller, PsyD, Emma C. Gilchrist, MPH, Kaile M. Ross, MA, Shale L. Wong, MD, MSPH, Alexander Blount, EdD, C.J. Peek, PhD. Core Competencies for Behavioral Health Providers Working in Primary Care. Prepared from the Colorado Consensus Conference. February 2016.

Miller, Gilchrist, Ross, and Wong of the Eugene S. Farley, Jr. Health Policy Center, University of Colorado School of Medicine organized and led this project. Blount of Antioch University New England and University of Massachusetts served as consultant for behavioral health competencies and training. Peek of the University of Minnesota served as consultant to facilitate the consensus process and help synthesize the resulting content.

Appendix B

Core Competencies for Behavioral Health Providers Working in Primary Care

Contents

Acknowledgements 1

Preamble to the Competencies 2

Eight Competencies at a Glance 4

   1. Identify and assess behavioral health needs as part of a primary care team 5

   2. Engage and activate patients in their care 7

   3. Work as a primary care team member to create and implement care plans that address behavioral health factors 9

   4. Help observe and improve care team function and relationships 11

   5. Communicate effectively with other providers, staff, and patients 13

   6. Provide efficient and effective care delivery that meets the needs of the population of the primary care setting 15

   7. Provide culturally responsive, whole-person and family-oriented care 17

   8. Understand, value, and adapt to the diverse professional cultures of an integrated care team 19

References 21

Appendix A. Colorado Consensus Conference Participants 22

Appendix B

Core Competencies for Behavioral Health Providers Working in Primary Care

Acknowledgements

The authors gratefully acknowledge the financial backing of the following foundations:
- The Colorado Health Foundation
- Caring for Colorado Foundation
- The Ben and Lucy Ana Walton Fund of the Walton Family Foundation
- Rose Community Foundation
- The Piton Foundation at Gary Community Investments

The authors also wish to thank the Colorado State Innovation Model leadership for their support, Linda Niebauer and Larry Green for their help in planning the Colorado Consensus Conference and final product development, and the Colorado Consensus Conference participants (see appendix A) for their time and feedback to improve the competencies.

Core Competencies for Behavioral Health Providers Working in Primary Care

Preamble to the Competencies

Consensus on the eight core competencies for licensed behavioral health providers working in primary care was established at the Colorado Consensus Conference on November 17, 2015, with revisions called for at that meeting and subsequently reviewed by the participant group in December of 2015. This preamble sets the stage for understanding the eight competencies.

Competence as a licensed behavioral health provider working in primary care refers to the *knowledge, skills, and attitudes*—and their interconnectedness—that allow an individual to perform the tasks and roles in that setting (adapted from Kaslow, Dunn, & Smith, 2008). These competencies are completely compatible with the five generic core competencies for healthcare professionals as articulated in the 2003 Institute of Medicine report, *Health Professions Education: A Bridge to Quality*. The goal for all members of the primary care team is to acquire and demonstrate competencies specific to their roles in integrated primary care. The scope of this document is the desired competencies tailored for licensed behavioral health providers.

General Definition of Integrated Behavioral Health

The competencies relate to the Agency for Healthcare Research and Quality (AHRQ) definition of integrated behavioral health and primary care:

> "The care a patient experiences as a result of a team of primary care and behavioral health clinicians, working together with patients and families, using a systematic and cost-effective approach to provide patient-centered care for a defined population.
>
> This care may address mental health and substance use conditions, health behaviors (including their contribution to chronic medical illnesses), life stressors and crises, stress-related physical symptoms, and ineffective patterns of healthcare utilization." Peek, C.J. and the National Integration Academy Council (2013)

Cross-Cutting Themes for the Eight Competencies

Several repeating themes were identified that apply across all of the competencies. Rather than repeating them within each of the eight competencies, which leads to long, repetitive-sounding competency descriptions, these cross-cutting themes or tenets are listed here once as applying across all the competencies.

The behavioral health provider competencies are written to apply broadly:

- Across a continuum from prevention to illness: to address prevention, wellness, mental health and substance use treatment, recovery, trauma, and quality of life
- Across the lifespan: from birth to end of life care
- Across the generations: children and elders in families or intergenerational relationships (that may involve guardians, family caregivers, or others), not only as individuals apart from such relationships
- Across a biopsychosocial continuum: integrating biological, psychological, social, and spiritual information and perspectives in evaluation and treatment
- Person-centered and culturally sensitive: tailoring care to patient values and preferences, culture and community, socioeconomics and health disparities, and religious, gender, sexual orientation or other important identifications

Core Competencies for Behavioral Health Providers Working in Primary Care

The Competencies Are Not Written for Any Particular Model or Type of Integration

Different clinics may employ different types of spatial arrangement, team structure, or styles of collaboration—sometimes known as "models," such as "co-location," "full-integration," "primary care behavioral health," or "collaborative care." These are often chosen on the basis of goals, stage of development, or what clinics find practical at any given time.

The eight competences are written to support highly integrated practices with on-site behavioral health providers as members of the primary care team. Practices will vary in how they implement or carry out these competencies, depending not only on their "model" of integration, but on their patient population, spatial arrangement, and operational support. For example, some competencies may be used more routinely or intensively depending on the type of collaboration or integration being used in practice and patient populations involved. In addition, these competencies do not take into account the additional elements needed for successful integration at the practice level (e.g., electronic medical records, workflow, spatial arrangements, and competencies for integrated care necessary for other team members). Such "model" characterizations can be found in the AHRQ Lexicon and SAMHSA/HRSA CIHS

The Competencies Are Specific to Behavioral Health Practice in Primary Care

These competencies do not attempt to re-create the entire scope of competencies for licensed behavioral health providers acquired in their basic training—only those *specific* to working *on a team in primary care* that may or may not stand out beyond those expected of licensed behavioral health providers in general.

Some competencies are learned through education in classes or on the job, while these and others may be developed and mastered as the behavioral health provider acquires experience in an integrated primary care setting.

How to Read the Competencies

The eight competencies are written at three levels of detail:

1. *Competency name with a one- or two-sentence description*: a title and high-level statement of what is included in the competency
2. *Bullet point list with headings*: this "unpacks" the high level description with specifics
3. *Examples of what you might see in action*: concrete and practical examples—"what you actually do"—adapted from the publications from which the eight competencies were originally drawn.

The Competencies Are Expected to Evolve Over Time

These are not offered as a final product for all time, but as a consensus starting point created among stakeholders on November 17, 2015, that can evolve through application in the field.

Abbreviations Used

behavioral health	BH	primary care provider	PCP
mental health	MH	electronic health record	EHR
substance abuse/use	SA		

Core Competencies for Behavioral Health Providers Working in Primary Care

Eight Competencies at a Glance

1. **Identify and assess behavioral health needs as part of a primary care team**
   BH providers apply knowledge of cognitive, emotional, biological, behavioral, and social aspects of health, MH, and medical conditions across the lifespan; and incorporate their clinical observations into an overall, team-based primary care assessment that may include identifying, screening, assessing, and diagnosing.

2. **Engage and activate patients in their care**
   BH providers engage patients in their care, helping them understand how their BH factors affect their health and illness, and how the BH aspects can be integrated in a team-based care plan.

3. **Work as a primary care team member to create and implement care plans that address behavioral health factors**
   BH providers work as members of the primary care team to collaboratively create and implement care plans that address BH factors in primary care practice. These factors may include mental illness, substance use disorders, and physical health problems requiring psychosocial interventions.

4. **Help observe and improve care team function and relationships**
   BH providers help the primary care team monitor and improve care team function and collaborative relationships. By knowing their own and others' roles, they help the team pool knowledge and experience to inform treatment, engage in shared decision-making with each other and with patients, and share responsibility for care and outcomes.

5. **Communicate effectively with other providers, staff, and patients**
   BH providers in primary care communicate effectively with providers, patients, and the primary care team with a willingness to initiate patient or family contact outside routine face-to-face clinical work. BH providers communicate in ways that build patient understanding, satisfaction, and the ability to participate in care.

6. **Provide efficient and effective care delivery that meets the needs of the population of the primary care setting**
   BH providers in primary care use their available time and effort on behalf of the practice population, setting prioritized agendas (with roles and goals) with patients and the team, managing brief and longer patient encounters effectively, and identifying areas for immediate and future work with appropriate follow-up care for which BH availability is maintained.

7. **Provide culturally responsive, whole-person and family-oriented care**
   BH providers in primary care employ the biopsychosocial model – approaching healthcare from biological, psychological, social, spiritual, and cultural aspects of whole-person care, including patient and family beliefs, values, culture, and preferences.

8. **Understand, value, and adapt to the diverse professional cultures of an integrated care team**
   BH providers act in ways consistent with the collaborative culture and mission of primary care with an attitude of flexibility. BH providers adapt their work style to meet patient needs while building confidence and comfort in working in primary care culture, with providers, and medical situations.

Core Competencies for Behavioral Health Providers Working in Primary Care

1. Identify and assess behavioral health needs as part of a primary care team

BH providers apply knowledge of cognitive, emotional, biological, behavioral, and social aspects of health, mental health, and medical conditions across the lifespan; and incorporate their clinical observations into an overall, team-based primary care assessment that may include identifying, screening, assessing, and diagnosing:

a. Mental illnesses, SA disorders, and adverse health behaviors commonly encountered in primary care —and the ways these often present in primary care practice
b. BH or psychosocial contributors to common physical health problems such as chronic illnesses and medically unexplained or stress-related physical symptoms
c. Complicated, unusual, or high-risk clinical situations with significant BH and social factors intertwined with medical care and/or barriers to care and patient self-management, using a broad range of information in medical record and PCP knowledge of patient history
d. Children, adolescents, and families with, or at risk for, psychosocial problems, further assessing:
   - Developmental problems and milestones
   - Potentially difficult situations in childcare, including bedtime, toileting, and feeding
   - Learning difficulties and attention deficit hyperactivity disorder
   - Psychosocial and environmental risk factors and stressors such as parental MH or family systems problems, adverse childhood experiences, and contextual factors affecting health and care such as home and school environments
   - How family, guardians, or caregivers can be part of overall care or health of the child, including potential parent training or coaching
e. Severe or persistent BH problems or psychiatric emergencies that require the assistance of specialized BH providers, services, or community-based resources

Identification (and targeted BH screening) in the areas above may be focused on identifying either populations or individuals with BH needs, and may use practice-level and claims data to assist in such identification.

Core Competencies for Behavioral Health Providers Working in Primary Care

Examples of "identify and assess" from McDaniel, et al., 2014:

- Identify behavioral or psychological factors in common primary care medical conditions (e.g., depression comorbid with diabetes and how blood sugar levels may affect cognition and mood)
- Interview effectively to identify problem, degree of functional impairment, and symptoms
- Conduct a suicide assessment on all patients identified with depressed mood
- Identify severe or treatment-resistant MH problems for triage to specialty MH, as available (e.g., psychotic and delusional disorders, complex trauma, severe personality disorders, eating disorders)
- Recognize names and purposes of medications for common medical and behavioral conditions (e.g., diabetes, hypertension, and depression) seen in primary care and the common side effects affecting mood or cognition
- Find out about support systems, spiritual resources, and connections to community resources
- Obtain information from caregivers and parents in the assessment process (e.g., help a caretaker identify health risks for a child with asthma residing with a smoker, and engage the parents in a conversation about change)
- Interview for health beliefs/attitudes that influence patient or family view of health, illness, and help-seeking
- Identify cognitive and emotional factors that influence a patient's or family's reaction to medical diagnoses, use of health information, and influence reactions to diagnoses, injury, and disability
- Recognize the effect of acute and chronic illness on physical and mental health of caregivers, parents, siblings, and other family members
- Assist primary care team in selecting measures to identify common problems (e.g., depression, anxiety, SA, sleep difficulties, disruptive child or adult behavior), and understand strengths and limitations of screening tools

Examples from Strosahl, 2005:

- Identify problems quickly and incorporate the patient's point-of-view
- Apply patient's strengths and resources to identified problems; focus on functional outcomes
- Evaluate readiness-to-change, and emphasize patient-driven change

Examples from CIHS, 2014:

- Recognize signs, symptoms and treatments of the most common health conditions, crises, and comorbidities seen in the healthcare setting
- Assess the family and social support system and other socioeconomic resources that can impact health and care

Core Competencies for Behavioral Health Providers Working in Primary Care

2. Engage and activate patients in their care

BH providers engage patients in their care, helping them understand how their BH factors affect their health and illness, and how the BH aspects can be integrated in a team-based care plan.

a. Use strong interpersonal skills to help patients feel comfortable and motivated, and to help the patient build a therapeutic relationship with the BH provider and primary care team by using language and an approach that helps overcome barriers or stigma to access BH services.
b. Involve care managers or other team members when appropriate to help patients and families engage fully in their care.
c. Explain the "why and how" of integrated care:
   - Educate patients about the conditions and BH factors in their clinical situation and care involving parents, families, guardians, or caregivers as appropriate to age and situation
   - Help patients understand and work with the primary care team and plan that includes BH, while addressing any discomfort with their care or barriers to it; using language to introduce BH providers that helps address the patient's confusion or fears
   - Triage patients to the appropriate level of care while managing the patient's needs in the interim
d. Engage patients and families in planning and decision-making regarding their care (see competency 4). In particular, engage patients in a manner consistent with their health literacy:
   - Engage patients at times when patients need to understand their choices and take an active role to the extent they wish
   - Engage patients and the team at times when there is a need to confirm a direction that is a good fit for the patient and the team—a plan that the patient understands and embraces
e. Set reasonable care team expectations, provide follow-up support for the patient, and promote care team transparency with the patient:
   - Work with primary care colleagues to help set realistic expectations of patient engagement in care (e.g., in which areas, if any, a patient is ready to participate, competing demands in their larger life context, realistic timeframes for developing patient readiness, and how pushing something prematurely may generate resistance)
   - Provide follow-up support for the patient, including connecting the patient to appropriate resources within the clinic and within their community
   - Use practice routines transparent to the patient (e.g., have team conversations about the patient in the presence of the patient, and facilitate patient access to records and notes)

Core Competencies for Behavioral Health Providers Working in Primary Care

Examples of "engage and activate patients" from McDaniel, et al, 2014:

- Engage the broader team by co-interviewing a patient with diabetes with a dietician
- Work with the pediatrician and respiratory therapist in a joint effort to develop a plan to improve a child's adherence to an asthma treatment regimen

Examples from Strosahl, 2005:

- Apply patient or family strengths and resources to identified problems
- Evaluate readiness-to-change, and emphasize patient-driven change

Examples from CIHS, 2014:

- Establish rapport and rapidly develop and maintain effective working relationships with diverse individuals, including healthcare consumers, family members, and other providers
- Listen actively and effectively—quickly grasp presenting problems, needs, and preferences as communicated by others and reiterate to ensure that it has been accurately understood
- Convey relevant information in a non-judgmental manner about BH, general health, and health behaviors using terms free of jargon and acronyms, and easily understood by the listener
- Explain to the patient and family the roles and responsibilities of each team member and how all will work together to provide services

Core Competencies for Behavioral Health Providers Working in Primary Care

3. Work as a primary care team member to create and implement care plans[1] that address behavioral health factors

BH providers work as members of the primary care team to collaboratively create and implement care plans that address BH factors in primary care practice. These factors may include mental illness, substance use disorders, and physical health problems requiring psychosocial interventions.

a. Work from a recognized role to identify, assess, educate, and treat as a member of the primary care team. This involves appropriate division of responsibility within the care team to help form care plans and carry out interventions that address the common clinical challenges (listed below—see competencies 1 and 2 for similar specifics reiterated here):
   - Mental illnesses and SA disorders
   - Physical health problems requiring psychosocial interventions in the care plan, e.g., BH contributors to a wide range of primary care presentations such as common chronic illnesses (e.g., asthma, diabetes, heart disease, irritable bowel syndrome, childhood illnesses), and medically unexplained physical symptoms
   - Complicated or high-risk cases with BH and social factors at the root of the risk or complexity
   - Adverse health behaviors commonly seen in primary care, along with associated prevention and health promotion strategies

b. Bring particular BH knowledge and skill to bear, such as:
   - Knowledge of human development to tailor BH services to patients across the lifespan
   - Influence of family systems, trauma or adverse childhood experiences on care and health, along with strategies to consider within care plans
   - Early identification and intervention for children and others with symptoms or risks who may not have a diagnosable condition
   - General knowledge of how psychosocial and BH factors and conditions interact with common primary care problems
   - Recognition of when a BH problem is outside the scope of primary care and needs other levels or types of care
   - Prevention, wellness, and health behavior interventions, e.g., sleep, parenting, healthy eating and exercise, self-regulation
   - Community resources, schools, agencies, home-based care programs

c. Help the primary care team negotiate care plans that are understood and embraced by patients, families, and caregivers, e.g., with:
   - Conversations and plans consistent with their health literacy
   - Shared treatment decisions that result in patients understanding their choices, and taking an active role to the extent they wish
   - A clinical team leader identified for each patient, based on the needs of the patient, and matching those needs with provider scope of practice, and relationship with the patient
   - Community resources to be mobilized in support of the care plan or self-management support
   - Sufficient patient/family confidence in ability to carry out the patient's role in treatment or health behavior change

d. Help the primary care team monitor patient progress on BH factors in care to ensure that the level of treatment provided in primary care is resolving symptoms.
   - Employ other or higher levels of care, as appropriate, based on monitored outcomes
   - Use data to help monitor progress, e.g., practice-level data such as registries, EHR, appointments, referrals along with claims data (if available), to help monitor and identify the need to adjust care plans that are not working

Core Competencies for Behavioral Health Providers Working in Primary Care

[1] Elements likely found in care plans involving integrated BH (excerpted from AHRQ Lexicon)

1. Team roles and goals—specific goals and team members responsible for specific goals or tasks.
2. Documentation of dialogue with the patient on why a shared record is an important component—the benefits (and any risks) to the patient—with exploration of any patient concerns about shared records and any precautions taken to protect the confidentiality of BH information.
3. Patient education about their conditions, treatments, and self-management.
4. Medical treatments, including pharmacologic treatment, a single shared medication list, and problem list.
5. Psychotherapy, community groups, or other non-pharmacologic BH or substance use therapy or support.
6. Counseling or coaching, e.g., motivational interviewing and behavioral activation.
7. How plan is tailored to patient/family context, e.g., cultural groups, language, schools, vocational, and community.
8. Expectation for implementation:
   - All involved providers read and work from the care plan—these are shared care plans
   - Likely indicators that improvement has begun are listed, along with who is most likely to notice the change first
   - Likely indicators that the care plan isn't working and may need to be revised, along with who should be informed that the care plan needs changing

Examples of "create and implement care plans" from McDaniel, et al., 2014:

Generalist skills:
- Use interventions to improve function in areas such as school and work responsibilities, improving quality of social interactions, decreasing disruptive behaviors, improving sleep, decreasing pain, reducing anxiety, improving mood and improving exercise and nutrition
- Implement evidence-based interventions (e.g., cognitive behavior therapy, parent–child interaction therapy, motivational interviewing, family psychoeducation, and problem-solving therapy)
- Offer interventions for patient self-care, symptom reduction, and functional improvement--with self-regulation such as deep breathing, relaxation, sleep hygiene, increased exercise, problem solving, and assertive communication
- Employ methods such as "Teach Back" to assure patient understanding of healthcare plans, and the patient's role in his/her own care
- Bridge appropriately among behavioral services offered in primary care and specialty MH and community resources
- Assist the primary care team on when and how to incorporate integrated BH provider into the care process
- Help primary care team engage challenging patients in a manner that enhances care, e.g., BH provider readily available to primary care team to discuss ways to interact effectively with patients or families with challenging interpersonal styles and complicated medical or social situations

Common chronic illness:
- Plan care that takes into account relevant factors (physical, behavioral, cognitive, environmental, and social) that can affect pain (for example), and considering health literacy level and cultural beliefs so as to engage patients in care for chronic pain beyond medication
- Offer interventions that include the family system, e.g., involve spouse or parents in nutritional planning for a patient with diabetes
- Provide psychoeducation and supportive counseling to family caregivers or parents of a patient or child with a particular condition

Biologic components/interactions:
- Describe the actions taken while working with the PCP that help engage patients with medically unexplained symptoms in regular care

Core Competencies for Behavioral Health Providers Working in Primary Care

4. Help observe and improve care team function and relationships[2]

BH providers help the primary care team monitor and improve care team function and collaborative relationships. By knowing their own and others' roles, they help the team pool knowledge and experience to inform treatment, engage in shared decision-making with each other and with patients, and share responsibility for care and outcomes.

   a. Know their own roles, contributions, and scope-of-practice (along with that of the other team members).
   b. Be flexible in role and work style to best fit the needs of the patients and team members.
   c. Help develop ways in which PCPs can introduce the BH provider that readily engage the patient and identify the BH provider as part of the care team, and clarify the kinds of situations for which the BH provider can be helpful with the clinic population.
   d. Help the team pool the knowledge and experience of all members (and their patients) to inform and enhance treatment.
   e. Use clinic-level data to help the team pool their knowledge to improve identification, plan care, evaluate efforts, and enhance integration strategies among the care team.
   f. Help the primary care team (along with other team members) identify and respond to problems in teamwork and collaboration, and to further develop the team functions.
   g. Share responsibility with PCPs for patient care and experience, total health outcomes, and cost/resource use (Triple Aim, Berwick et al, 2008).
   h. Participate in process improvement methods to enhance teamwork and clinical care.

[2] Care team function and relationships are often referred to as "inter-professional practice" because the teams are often comprised not only of PCPs and BH providers, but other professionals as well. These providers are to function as one team, rather than as "add-ons" who function more or less separately.

Core Competencies for Behavioral Health Providers Working in Primary Care

Examples of "help monitor and improve teamwork" from McDaniel et al, 2014:

- Promote effective collaborative decision-making in care teams, including the facilitation of team members communicating their own observations and perspectives
- Regard patient care as the responsibility of a team of professionals, not that of a single provider
- Consider the patient/parents/family to be key members of the healthcare team—who also need to understand team roles and functions. Recognize, respect, and support activities of other primary care team members to provide BH services—it is not all up to the BH provider
- Clarify the various roles of the BH provider to team members, recognizing when and how to use other team members' specific disciplinary expertise
- Give PCPs actionable recommendations that are brief, concrete, and evidence-based
- Provide immediate (e.g., same day) brief, feedback to a consulting PCP, avoiding psychological jargon
- Convey and receive both urgent and routine clinical information to primary care team members, using appropriate infrastructure (e.g., face-to-face, phone, e-mail, EHR tasks, consults, and chart notes)
- Lead or participate in staff, clinical, and organizational meetings.
- Work with clinical leaders and care team to design, implement, and evaluate quality improvement initiatives regarding integrated BH

Examples from Strosahl, 2005:

- Distinguish between a consultation/teamwork model and an individual psychotherapy model
- Explain the team role of the BH provider accurately to the patient, parent, or family
- Operate comfortably within the primary care extended team culture
- Frequently circulate through the medical practice area to create top-of-mind awareness among primary care team members
- Readily provide unscheduled services when needed
- Be available for on-demand consultations by pager or cellphone

Examples from CIHS, 2014:

- Recognize, respect and value the role and expertise of patients, family members, BH providers, and PCPs
- Serve as a member of an inter-professional team, helping other members quickly conceptualize a patient's strengths, problems, and appropriate plan of care
- Foster shared decision-making with patients, family members, and other providers
- Demonstrate practicality, flexibility, and adaptability in working with others, emphasizing the achievement of treatment goals as opposed to rigid adherence to treatment models

Core Competencies for Behavioral Health Providers Working in Primary Care

5. Communicate effectively with other providers, staff, and patients

BH providers in primary care use their available time and effort on behalf of the practice population, setting prioritized agendas (with roles and goals) with patients and the team, managing brief and longer patient encounters effectively, and identifying areas for immediate and future work with appropriate follow-up care for which BH availability is maintained, such as:

a. Communicate frequently with (and facilitate communication among) PCPs, BH providers, and other team members. "Frequent" is a large part of "effective." Other aspects of "effective" include being clear, concise, timely, and relevant to the situation at hand and in language others can readily understand. (See competency 8 for additional information).
b. Contact patients/families outside of face-to-face clinical work, as needed, in accordance with practice policies and patient/family preferences, e.g., brief calls, approved forms of email, texts, etc.
c. Facilitate communication among providers and between providers and patients in ways that increase transparency and build patient understanding, satisfaction, and ability to participate in care. Examples include:

- Weekly or other regular team meetings regarding patient care
- Brief daily meetings, "huddles," or case reviews
- "Warm handoffs" between providers and patients
- "Curbside consultations" between providers—including communication and teamwork issues
- Consultations about patients for whom the BH provider is not (or will not be) providing direct care, e.g., consulting or coaching a PCP on a clinical question
- Telephone follow-ups with patients or other providers
- BH connections in the medical neighborhood with outside providers, case managers, specialists, community-based people who are involved with the patient or family but not part of the clinic team, etc.
- Formal communications, e.g., case presentations that serve as vehicles for communication, consultation, or education

d. Communicate with primary care colleagues in a professional and ethical manner consistent with the medical culture or methods that enhance the integrated care delivery. (For more, see competency 8.)
e. Be aware of the broad range of needs for communication tailored to the situation, e.g., regarding individual patients, populations or panels of patients, high-risk or high-cost situations, care coordination, specialty providers, and community organizations.
f. Communicating through documentation and shared health records in a manner accessible and clear to the rest of the integrated team and to patients.

Core Competencies for Behavioral Health Providers Working in Primary Care

Examples of "communicate effectively" from McDaniel et al., 2014:

- Proactively help team members better understand their interpersonal and communication styles, and how to work together more effectively
- Communicate effectively with team members and patients or families in a manner that is sensitive to power differentials present in a clinical setting
- Facilitate team process when there are professional disagreements by focusing on shared goals
- Use systems thinking and relationship skills typical of BH providers to address malfunctioning team behavior
- Write clear, concise EHR notes with key information and short, specific recommendations and plan
- Ensure EHR notes are accessible to the primary care team, knowing they may be accessible to the patient
- Encourage patients and families to use the patient portal of the EHR

Examples from Strosahl, 2005:

- Provide feedback to referring providers on the same day when there is a consultation question
- Tailor team recommendations at the pace and flow of the medical clinic
- Conduct effective curbside consultations
- Give recommendations that are concrete and easily understood by all primary care team members
- Write clear, concise chart notes indicating BH treatment plan, treatment response, and patient adherence to self-management—protecting sensitive and confidential information.
- Be knowledgeable of mandated reporting requirements on abuse and neglect

Core Competencies for Behavioral Health Providers Working in Primary Care

6. Provide efficient and effective care delivery that meets the needs of the population of the primary care setting

BH providers in primary care use their available time and effort on behalf of the practice population, setting prioritized agendas (with roles and goals) with patients and the team, managing brief (as well as longer) patient encounters effectively, and identifying areas for immediate and future work with appropriate follow-up care for which BH availability is maintained.

Key distinctions to be mastered:

- *Clinic panel vs. caseload*: BH provider's time in primary care is focused on serving the entire clinic panel consistent with "panel (or population) management". In some cases this focus may be on a designated subpopulation (e.g., diabetes and depression). In either case, the BH provider's time is focused on serving an identified population rather than only on patients who happen to find their way onto a BH provider's "caseload."
    - Primary care practices may define their practice panels differently, and hence the patient population for BH providers may differ (e.g., the boundary practices set between primary care and specialty care or whether to provide complete care for patients with serious and persistent MH or SA problems). Clinics may decide to focus their BH on a subset of its total population, e.g., children with special needs, SA, depression, high risk or chronically ill, "super-utilizers," or other such subset. The "population" that the BH provider will care for will depend on how the clinic defines its population or target sub-population for BH integration.

- *Efficient and effective*: There is no such thing as efficient care that is ineffective; therefore, efficient doesn't mean merely "fast" or "short." "Efficient and effective" means care is clinically effective at the same time it is done with a minimum of wasted motion, rework, delay, or cumbersome method. Analogy: "Concise" means all the necessary information with no wasted words. This competency is about "concise" in this sense – not only about time spent, but including time spent.

- *Brief vs. long visits*: The "right" appointment length depends on what the patient needs at that time—and can range from a 5-minute introduction or warm handoff to a 15- or 30-minute return visit for monitoring and coaching, to a 45- or 60-minute (or longer) evaluation visit. This competency involves flexibility to consciously match visit time to patient need, not to assume a "default" or habitual 50 minutes (or 15 minutes) for all visits.

- *Brief vs. longitudinal*: Much BH in primary care is done using brief, therapeutic approaches that fit the presenting problem and patient goals for progress with that problem. Mastery of such practical approaches is essential; however, in the primary care setting patients may return for care periodically over their lifespan rather than receiving one, short episode of BH care at the outset.

Examples of areas for effective-efficient practice management for BH providers:

a. Flexibility
  - Be available in person and by phone or email, interruptible, and willing to improvise in scheduling and how patient contact is made
  - Use physical space to increase visibility and presence in the midst of the primary care "traffic"

b. Know when to employ coordination, consultation, and collaboration (from Cohen et al, 2015)
  - Coordination:
    - Coordinate BH care with other providers whose care has similar goals but is being done more or less independently

Core Competencies for Behavioral Health Providers Working in Primary Care

- Steps may include contacting the other clinician, rapid briefing about patient situation and the issues to coordinate, and agreement on how to do so
- Know when to triage, refer, or navigate to specialties or community referral instead of coordinating with the primary care team

- Consultation:
  - Share information, diagnoses, and impressions with primary care team members that add to the pool of important information, while making efficient use of their time
  - Seek input/consultation from other providers with different expertise in ways that are succinct, and respect their workflows and sense of time while getting the needed consultation

- Collaboration:
  - Work jointly with PCPs and other team members to assess and develop care plans with patients and families
  - Ask for a consultation or initiate a change in care when the BH/team care isn't working

C. High-value use of appointment time

- Introduce self clearly and quickly, describing BH's role on the team and services available, to build rapport and orient patient to visit
- Identify problems, functional impairments, symptoms, patient concerns, and reason for referral early in initial visit. Summarize your understanding of problem(s) at appropriate level for patient and family, and check for accuracy.
- Further assess symptoms, BH concerns, other concerns, patient story, and family history, paying attention to:
  - Crisis assessment and triage—need for ongoing care and/or referrals to specialists and community resources
  - Use of screening or assessment tools, whether universal or targeted
  - Health behavior change, which may include prevention and early intervention
- Select appointment time and length, when possible, based on patient needs

Examples of "provide efficient and effective care" from McDaniel et al., 2014:

- Use appointment time efficiently (e.g., in a 30-minute appointment, identify problem(s), degree of functional impairment, and symptoms early in the visit)
- Summarize for patient and family or parents, when possible, an understanding of the problem (e.g., in 2–3 minutes) at the appropriate level, depth, and specificity for each patient in the context of their cultural beliefs

Examples from Strosahl, 2005:

- Use 30-minute sessions effectively
- Measure outcomes of behavior change or goals at every visit, developing alternative treatments when indicated
- Stay on time when conducting consecutive appointments
- Use community resource and social support strategies
- Use intermittent visit strategy to support home-based practice model/self-management
- Choreograph BH visits within existing medical services, appointments and processes
- Use flexible patient contact strategies, e.g., visits, phone, letter, email, and portals
- Coordinate triage of patients to and from external BH specialty services

Core Competencies for Behavioral Health Providers Working in Primary Care

7. Provide culturally responsive, whole-person and family-oriented care

BH providers in primary care employ the biopsychosocial model – approaching healthcare from biological, psychological, social, spiritual, and cultural aspects of whole-person care, including patient and family beliefs, values, culture, and preferences.

Use the biopsychosocial model treating health, illness, assessment, and care as the product of intertwined biological, psychological, and social factors (social determinants of health). Recognize and address these perspectives in whole-person care.

Note: Biological and psychological factors are described in competencies 1 and 3. This competency emphasizes culturally responsive, whole person care:

a. Social factors

- Take into account the role of social functioning and relationships in health, illness, health practices, health beliefs, and participation in treatment including economic and other barriers to care
- Take into account the role of social determinants of health, e.g., economic, socioeconomic status, and other barriers to health and care such as residential safety and stability, level of social/vocational connectedness, level of distress and distraction, level of trust in providers
- Identify and integrate individual, family, and cultural strengths in supportive patient care—making use of these assets, with family broadly defined to fit the patient's concept of his/her family
- Understand the impact of stigma related to BH problems. Work toward de-stigmatization of BH problems and treatment, using terminology that is appropriate to the culture of the patient and to the primary care setting where BH care is part of general healthcare
- Develop relationships with community organizations, agencies or schools that offer resources to more fully meet patients' needs, including non-medical resources addressing needs across the lifespan. Identify those with which the patient or family is already familiar or comfortable as part of their own community

b. Cultural and spiritual factors

- Take into account gender, gender identity, sexual orientation, disability, ethnicity/race, age, and other distinctive cultural or personal identifications while planning and providing care
- Tailor care plans to reported patient or family beliefs about health, illness, health practices, and how they are accustomed to participating in treatment (e.g., a refugee accustomed to specialist-based systems and work-ups)
- Quickly adapt treatment approaches based on cultural factors to help make care more acceptable or successful
- While planning and implementing care plans, use knowledge of health disparities to proactively address access, economic, and cultural factors such as language and any need for interpreters
- Inquire about and consider how spirituality and religion shapes the patient and family's responses to illness, care, and recovery

Core Competencies for Behavioral Health Providers Working in Primary Care

Examples of "culturally responsive, whole person care" from McDaniel et al., 2014:

- Ask patients, families, and team members about cultural identities, health beliefs, and illness history that affect health behaviors
- Demonstrate sensitivity to a variety of factors that influence healthcare (e.g., developmental, cultural, socioeconomic, religious, sexual orientation)
- Modify interventions for BH change in response to social and cultural factors
- Use culturally sensitive measures and procedures when conducting research, evaluation or quality improvement projects
- Help patients communicate with healthcare professionals who have cultural backgrounds different from their own (and vice-versa)
- Use language appropriate to the patient's education and culture
- Recognize the relationships among ethnicity, race, gender, age/cohort, religion, sexual orientation, culture, disability, and health behavior in primary care
- Engage schools, community agencies, or healthcare systems (that the patient or family can relate to) that support patient care and function

Examples from CIHS, 2014:

- Use the primary language and preferred mode of communication of the patient and family members or communicate through the use of qualified interpreters
- Adapt style of communication to ensure a patient's ability to process and understand information
- Provide health education materials appropriate to the communication style and literacy of the patient and family, and that reinforce information provided verbally during healthcare visits
- Recognize and manage personal biases related to patients, families, health conditions and healthcare delivery

Appendix B

Core Competencies for Behavioral Health Providers Working in Primary Care

8. Understand, value, and adapt to the diverse professional cultures of an integrated care team

BH providers act in ways consistent with the collaborative culture and mission of primary care with an attitude of flexibility. BH providers adapt their work style to meet patient needs while building confidence and comfort in working in primary care culture, with providers, and medical situations.

Note: Much of this is implicit in other competencies, but is brought together here explicitly for the benefit of the entire primary care team, including the BH providers.

a. Evolve and reinforce values and attitudes consistent with the team-based culture and population health mission of primary care and the role of BH providers in it, modifying personal habits or behavior accordingly

- Cite evidence for the value of incorporating BH services into primary care to patients, families, and providers when it proves useful
- Develop comfort and confidence in working with PCPs and in medical situations, adopting an attitude of flexibility; and adapting work content and style as needed to serve the best interest of patients, parents, families, or the patient's caregivers
- Ensure with the primary care team that high patient care volume is accompanied by tools and methods to provide quality BH care to populations and individuals, e.g., tools to track high-risk patients until stabilized or engaged in higher level of care
- Understand the local organizational mission, structure, and historical factors supporting the role of BH providers in integrated care

b. Understand and respect different team roles and scope of practice

- Communicate BH providers' professional scope of practice (and limitations) in context of the primary care team and across the patient lifespan
- Know the particular roles, values, cultures, scope of practice, and expertise of each team member so that trust and ability to depend on each other is enhanced by mutual understanding among physicians, nurse practitioners, physician assistants, BH providers, care managers, pharmacists, nurses, social workers, or others on the practice or extended team

c. Recognize ethical issues and code of conduct values across the primary care team

- Recognize and manage the ethical issues common in integrated care and primary care in general, including differences and similarities in concepts of confidentiality for BH in the team-based primary care setting and specialty MH settings
- Acknowledge and become familiar with the various codes of ethics and conduct among different disciplines on the healthcare team, including the common themes and differences
- Adhere to the code of ethics, conduct, and licensure of your particular discipline with an awareness of how these may or may not be applied differently in different work settings such as MH clinics, primary care clinics, hospitals or community organizations
- Practice appropriate documentation and business practices such as credentialing

Core Competencies for Behavioral Health Providers Working in Primary Care

Examples of "understand and adapt to diverse professional cultures" from McDaniel et al., 2014:

- Convey to other team members and patients the typical roles, skills and activities of BH providers in primary care across populations such as children, adults, and elderly
- Adapt role and activities in the best interest of patient care (e.g., serving as treating provider, consultant, team leader, advocate, care manager, health educator, or community liaison—depending on situation and need)
- Participate in professional or other learning groups on integrated BH as a professional activity
- Demonstrate a commitment to ethical principles regarding dual relationships, confidentiality, informed consent, boundary issues, team functioning, and others
- Manage stress associated with primary care practice via a consultation network with other integrated BH providers
- Evaluate own competencies and determine need for continuing education
- Act in best interest of the patient by seeking consultation or professional support in situations when needed
- Make use of supervisory or peer consultation support for BH providers within the organization
- Practice appropriate documentation, billing, and reimbursement procedures
- Follow laws on abuse reporting, adolescent reproductive health, and determination of decision-making capacity
- Demonstrate familiarity with hospital/medical setting bylaws, credentialing, privileges, and staffing responsibilities, and standards set forth by national accrediting bodies
- Engage the organization and its leaders at key times in making change that promotes integrated BH and ensure necessary resources for effective integrated BH practice

Core Competencies for Behavioral Health Providers Working in Primary Care

References

General definitions of competency:

Kaslow, N. J., Dunn, S. E., & Smith, C. O. (2008). Competencies for psychologists in academic health centers (AHCs). *Journal of Clinical Psychology in Medical Settings*, 15, 18–27. doi:10.1007/s10880-008-9094-y

Institute of Medicine (2003). The Core Competencies Needed for Health Care Professionals. IOM Committee on the Health Professions Education Summit; Greiner AC, Knebel E, editors. *Health Professions Education: A Bridge to Quality. Washington (DC);* National Academies Press. Available from: http://www.ncbi.nlm.nih.gov/books/NBK221519/

Core Competencies for Collaborative Practice (2011). Report of an expert panel sponsored by the *Interprofessional Education Collaborative* that consists of organizations from nursing, medicine, pharmacy, dental, medical colleges, and schools of public health. http://www.aacn.nche.edu/education-resources/ipecreport.pdf

General definition of integrated behavioral health excerpted from:

Peek, C.J. and the National Integration Academy Council (2013). Lexicon for Behavioral Health and Primary Care Integration: Concepts and Definitions Developed by Expert Consensus". *Agency for Healthcare Research and Quality*, Rockville MD. http://integrationacademy.ahrq.gov/lexicon

Main competency statements adapted from:

Kinman CR, Gilchrist EC, Payne-Murphy JC, Miller BF. Provider- and practice-level competencies for integrated behavioral health in primary care: a literature review. (Prepared by Westat under Contract No. HHSA 290-2009-00023I). Rockville, MD: Agency for Healthcare Research and Quality. March 2015.
http://integrationacademy.ahrq.gov/sites/default/files/AHRQ_AcadLitReview.pdf

Specific examples or behaviors drawn or adapted from:

McDaniel SH, Grus CL, Cubic BA, Hunter CL, Kearney LK, Schuman CC, Karel MJ, Kessler RS, Larkin KT, McCutcheon S, Miller BF (2014). Competencies for psychology practice in primary care. *American Psychologist*. 69(4):409.

Strosahl K. (2005). Training behavioral health and primary care providers for integrated care: A core competencies approach. Chapter in *Behavioral Integrative Care: Treatments That Work in the Primary Care Setting*., pp. 53-71. W. O'Donohue, M. Byrd, N. Cummings, & D. Henderson (eds). New York: Brunner-Routledge

Core competencies for integrated behavioral health and primary care; *Center for Integrated Health Solutions (CIHS); SAMHSA-HRSA and National Council for Behavioral Health*. www.integration.samhsa.gov

Other references

Berwick DM, Nolan TW, Whittington J. The triple aim: care, health, and cost. Health Affairs. 2008 May 1;27(3):759-69.

Cohen DJ, Davis M, Balasubramanian BA, Gunn R, Hall J, Peek CJ, Green LA, Stange KC, Pallares C, Levy S, Pollack D. Integrating behavioral health and primary care: consulting, coordinating and collaborating among professionals. *The Journal of the American Board of Family Medicine*. 2015 Sep 1;28(Supplement 1):S21-31.

Core Competencies for Behavioral Health Providers Working in Primary Care

Appendix A. Colorado Consensus Conference Participants

Sarah Barnes, Colorado Children's Campaign
Alexander Blount, EdD, University of Massachusetts Medical School
Shandra Brown Levey, PhD, University of Colorado Department of Family Medicine
Adam Burstein, DO, Children's Hospital Colorado
JC Carrica, EdD, CAC, Southeast Health Group
Marceil Case, Health Care, Policy and Financing
Colleen Casper, RN, MS, DNP, Colorado Nursing Association
Colleen Church, MPA, Caring for Colorado Foundation
Maribel Cifuentes, RN, The Colorado Health Foundation
Whitney Connor, Rose Community Foundation
Laura Cote Gonzalez, PhD, Denver Health
Perry Dickinson, MD, University of Colorado Department of Family Medicine
Andrea Dwyer, Colorado School of Public Health
Caitlin Evrard, MPH, Colorado Department of Public Health and Environment
Jessica Fern, MPP, Colorado Health Institute
Emma Gilchrist, MPH, Eugene S. Farley, Jr. Health Policy Center
Stephanie Gold, MD, Eugene S. Farley, Jr. Health Policy Center
Kim Gorgens, PhD, ABPP, University of Denver
Larry Green, MD, Eugene S. Farley, Jr. Health Policy Center
Jennifer Grote, PhD, Denver Health
Patrece Hairston-Peetz, PsyD, Colorado Children's Healthcare Access Program
Emily Haller, BA, Colorado Behavioral Healthcare Council
William Heller, Colorado Department of Health Care, Policy and Financing
Aubrey Hill, Colorado Coalition for the Medically Underserved
Steve Holloway, Colorado Department of Public Health and Environment
Laurie Ivey, PsyD, Swedish Family Medicine Residency
Emily Johnson, Colorado Health Institute
Mita Johnson, Walden University!
Mindy Klowden, MNM, Jefferson Center for Mental Health
Kyle Knierim, MD, University of Colorado Department of Family Medicine
Marilyn Krajicek, EdD, RN, FAAN, CU College of Nursing
Erin Lantz, Colorado Community Health Network
Nadine Lund, BS, CPCC, Colorado Department of Public Health and Environment
Kevin Masters, PhD, University of Colorado Denver Department of Psychology
Lorez Meinhold, Keystone Policy Center
Mary Kay Meintzer, LPC, CACII, Sheridan Health Services
Benjamin Miller, PsyD, Eugene S. Farley Jr., Health Policy Center
Sam Monson, PsyD, Denver Health
Linda Niebauer, Eugene S. Farley, Jr. Health Policy Center
Sydney Oelerich, SIM Workforce Program Manager
Mike Olson, PhD, LMFT, St. Mary's Family Medicine Residency
Linda Osterland, PhD, Regis University
CJ Peek, PhD, University of Minnesota Medical School
Mark Queirolo, MPA, Colorado Department of Health Care Policy & Financing
Alex Reed, PsyD, MPH, University of Colorado Department of Family Medicine
Lenya Robinson, MA, LPC, Colorado Department of Health Care Policy and Financing
Kaile Ross, Eugene S. Farley, Jr. Health Policy Center
Don Sutton, PhD, Colorado Department of Public Health and Environment
Michael Talamantes, LCSW, University of Denver
Brian Turner, MPH, Colorado Behavioral Health Council

Core Competencies for Behavioral Health Providers Working in Primary Care

Patricia Uris, PhD, Colorado Department of Public Health and Environment
Alice Vienneau, LCSW, Denver Health
Robyn Wearner, MA, RD, University of Colorado Department of Family Medicine
Mary Weber, PhD, PMHNP-BC, University of Colorado College of Nursing
Tanya Weinberg, The Colorado Health Foundation
Shale Wong, MD, MSPH, Eugene S. Farley, Jr. Health Policy Center

Index

A
Accountable Care Organizations, 64
ADAPT approach, 207
Adaptive system, 106
Advanced alternative payment models (APMs), 197
Advancing Care Together (ACT), 4, 6, 48, 158, 159
Advocacy groups, behavioral health conditions, 199
Agency for Healthcare Research and Quality (AHRQ) Integration Academy, 13, 17, 85, 140, 160
Art of Critical Decision Making, 43
Atlas of Integrated Behavioral Health Care Quality Measures, 161

B
Balancing fidelity worksheet, 26–28
Behavioral health appointments, 72
Behavioral health clinicians (BHCs) training program, 47, 72, 133, 165, 166, 191
   hiring, 140–142
   Recruitment and Partnership, 76–81
   Referral Access Tool, 92
   Referral Request Policy, 92
   workflows, 145–148
Behavioral Health Consultant model, 137
Behavioral health insurance coverage with physical health coverage, 196
Behavioral health practice, 152
Behavioral health problems, 1, 3
Behavior Change Model, 90
Blended fee-for-service and capitation, 185
Bundled payments, 185
Business case preparation for integration, 189
Business model, 206

C
Centers for Medicaid and Medicare Services (CMS), 212
Chronic care model, 135
Clinical needs and business logistics, 63
Clinical priorities, 95
Clinical work, 104
Clinic financial health, 73

© Springer Nature Switzerland AG 2019
S. B. Gold, L. A. Green (eds.), *Integrated Behavioral Health in Primary Care*, https://doi.org/10.1007/978-3-319-98587-9

CMS billing codes for telehealth
services, 193
Cognitive-based therapy, 65
Collaborative care model
(CCM), 24–26, 65,
135–137, 188
Co-location, 133–135
Communication, team
functioning, 143–145
Community-Centered Medical
Home, 47
Community Mental Health
Center, 47, 48,
52, 71, 73
and primary care
providers, 78
Community Needs
Assessment, 78
Compact tool, 54, 55
Competitive business advantage
for employers, 40
Complex adaptive leadership,
105, 121, 125, 126
adaptive system, 110
clinical quality, 108
cockpit culture, 114
extensive onboarding, 113
flatten hierarchies, 114
flexibility, 119
formal therapy
office, 109
healthcare system, 112
heating system, 106
hiring process, 111
homeostasis, 107
implementation skills, 111
internal state
measurement, 107
measurement-based
management, 115
medical and psychosocial
attention, 118
patients' health care, 109
physical, psychological, social
and environmental
stressors, 121
physiologic limits/
parameters, 106
principles of, 116
productivity and patient
satisfaction, 108
quality improvement effort
for children, 120
reward interesting
solutions, 114
scheduling system, 110
support and promote
communication, 113
system transformation, 112
team based care, 112
training investment, 113
transformation effort,
122–124
uncertainty level, 107
vision/mission
statement, 109
workflow efficiency, 108
Comprehensive Primary Care
Plus Initiative, 197
Current Procedural Terminology
(CPT) codes, 187, 188

D

Data in quality improvement,
161, 170
Diagnostic and Statistical
Manual of Mental
Disorders-V
(DSM-V), 65
DIAMOND Initiative, 25

E

Electronic health record (EHR)
system, 159
Elevator Speech, 127, 128
Evidence-based protocol of
treatment, 135
Extension for Community
Healthcare Outcomes
(ECHO) model, 193

F

Family medicine residencies, 23
Fee-for-service, reimbursement, 185
Financial analysis, 48
Financial planning, nonrevenue gains, 67–68
  economic gains/increased revenue, 73
  economic losses/decreased revenue, 73
  objective and subjective measures, 75
  performance and productivity strategy, 74
  workforce salary data, 74
Financial sustainability, 63

G

Gantt chart, implementation timeline for behavioral health integration, 61, 62
General Behavioral Health Integration code, 188
Global payment/capitation, 186
Granular implementation, practice, 21
GROW pathway, 66
Guiding coalition, 41–45

H

Healing, transformational process, 41
Health and Behavior Assessment and Intervention codes, 187
Health care delivery, 186
Healthcare production factories, 104
Health-care quality, 158
Healthcare system, 106
  savings, 70
Health policy challenges, 178

I

Improving Access to Psychological Therapy program, 198
Integrated behavioral health, 206
Integrated care, 205
Integrating primary care and behavioral health, 205
Integration Project Organization, 97, 100
International Policy, 197, 198
Issue-specific organizations, 199

L

Language and communication, 53
Leadership, 207
  integration, 42
Licensed Clinical Social Workers (LCSWs), 191
Logic models, 97–99

M

Measurement principles, clinical care, 159, 160, 164
Medicaid and Medicare Innovation projects, 199
Medical and behavioral health, 53
  care, 207
Medical principles and contemporary core values, 36
Medicare Access and CHIP Reauthorization Act (MACRA), 197
Medicine
  contemporary values, 36
  foundational values, 36
  and primary care, 35
Mental health, prevalence, 1
Merit-based Incentive Payment System (MIPS), 197
Model of integration, 21, 24

N

National Committee for Quality Assurance (NCQA), 60, 212
National Institute for Health and Clinical Excellence (NICE) guidelines, 35
National Quality Forum (NQF) measures, 64
NCQA's Patient-Center Medical Home model, 38
Noneconomic gains
  in behavioral health integration, 69
  Quadruple Aim, 69

O

Operating models of behavioral health integration, 22–23
Optimal Healing Environment, 74
Organizational skills, collaborative team, 42
Outline evaluation metrics, 121

P

Patient-centered care, 35
Patient-centered medical home (PCMH) services, 39, 66, 92, 185
  principles of care and organizational needs, 49–51
Patient Health Questionnaire (PHQ)
  PHQ-2, 158
  PHQ-9, 168
Patient privacy and data sharing, 194–196
Pay for Performance (P4P) metrics, 185
Payment mechanisms, 178
Payment models for integrated behavioral health, 179–184
Payment policies, 211
Personal and conversational approach, 37
Personomics, 35
Physician champion/innovation team, 12
Policy change opportunities, 190, 193
Positional bargaining, 48
Practice transformation, 105, 212
Primary care, 46
Primary care behavioral health adaptation, 139
Primary Care Behavioral Health (PCBH) model of integration, 133, 137–139, 208
Primary care environment, 17–21
Primary care practice, 73
Primary care provider (PCP) practice, 122
Primary care-trained behavioral health clinicians, 191
Professional organizations, 199
Project-specific organizations, 199–200

Q

Quality of integrated care quality, 162–163

R

Reach, Effectiveness, Adoption, Implementation, and Maintenance (RE-AIM), 164–167, 211
Referral Access Tool, 92
Referral Request Policy, 92
Research methods, 4

Residency behavioral science education model, 23, 24
Right care, 35
Rule of thumb, 13

S

Screening, care process, 168
Shared-savings models, 71, 186
Social determinants of health, 35
Solution-Focused Brief Therapy (SFBT), 65, 66
SSRI, 148–150, 152, 209
Staff development and patient engagement, 81–86
Substance use disorders, 1

T

Team-based care, 7, 132
  rudimentary form, 38
TEAMCare, 65
Team culture, 142, 143
Team maintenance, 153

Telepsychiatry service, 47
Tracking tools, 170
Transforming primary care practices, 178

V

Value-based care payments, 71
Vice President of Corporate Business Development, 52
Vision and mission statements, 38–40

W

Westminster Medical Clinic (WMC), 34, 60, 74, 78, 94, 204
Whole-person care, 205, 212
Workflows and clinical outcomes, 87–96
Workforce challenges, 191, 192

Printed and bound by PG in the USA